Critical Muslim 37

Virus

Critical Muslim is published quarterly by C. Hurst & Co. (Publishers) Ltd. on behalf of and in conjunction with Critical Muslim Ltd. and the Muslim Institute, London.

All editorial correspondence to Muslim Institute, CAN Mezzanine, 49–51 East Road, London N1 6AH, United Kingdom.
E-mail: editorial@criticalmuslim.com

The editors do not necessarily agree with the opinions expressed by the contributors. We reserve the right to make such editorial changes as may be necessary to make submissions to *Critical Muslim* suitable for publication.

C. Hurst & Co (Publishers) Ltd., 41 Great Russell Street, London WC1B 3PL

ISBN: 978-1-78738-486-6 ISSN: 2048-8475

To subscribe or place an order by credit/debit card or cheque (pounds sterling only) please contact Kathleen May at the Hurst address above or e-mail kathleen@hurstpub.co.uk

Tel: 020 7255 2201

A one-year subscription, inclusive of postage (four issues), costs £50 (UK), £65 (Europe) and £75 (rest of the world), this includes full access to the *Critical Muslim* series and archive online. Digital only subscription is £3.30 per month.

A Cataloguing-in-Publication data record for this book is available from the British Library

CM37

WINTER 2021

CONTENTS

VIRUS

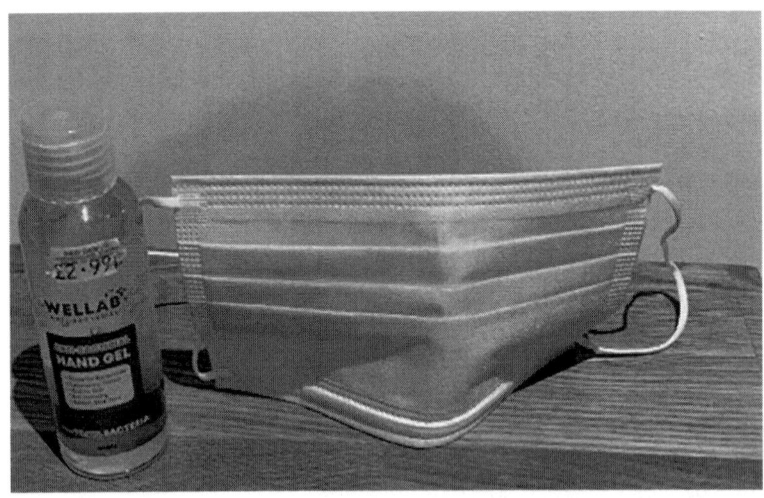

ARTS AND LETTERS

REVIEWS

ET CETERA

VIRUS

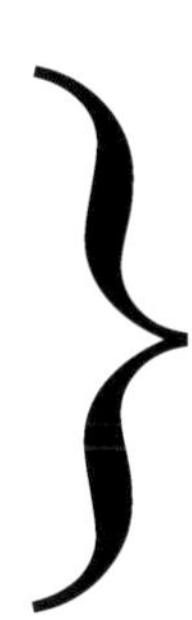

INTRODUCTION: VIRUS CHRONICLES *by Ehsan Masood*
JUSTICE FOR A PRAYING PERSON *by Anwar Ibrahim*
THE METAPHYSICS OF VIRUSES *by Colin Tudge*
FROM GOD TO GOD *by Syed Nomanul Haq*
QADAR *by Usama Hasan*
VIRAL CORONA CAPITALISM *by Vinay Lal*
MONTAGU AND OTTOMAN INOCULATION *by Iftikhar Malik*
COVID-19, ISLAM AND PSEUDOSCIENCE *by Nidhal Guessoum*
SWOLLEN FEET *by Chandrika Parmar*
IRANIAN DILEMMAS *by Lila Randall*
VIRAL DREAMS *by Leyla Jagiella*
EXISTENTIAL TERROR *by James Brooks*

INTRODUCTION: VIRUS CHRONICLES

Ehsan Masood

Michael Rosen is well known to millions of readers around the world, and to even more of their children, through his books of prose and poetry. Early in 2020, the much-loved writer, now 74, caught Covid-19. We know that older patients are particularly susceptible to the coronavirus, and for seven weeks Rosen was in intensive care at London's Whittington Hospital – six weeks breathing through a ventilator in an induced coma. His family thought at one point that they had lost him. He survived. But he has lost hearing in his left ear; his left eye is foggy, he has numbness in his toes, blood clots on his lungs and struggles with breathing.

The coronavirus pandemic of 2020 will have taken close to two million lives by the middle of 2021. It overwhelmingly kills older people with pre-existing medical conditions such as diabetes and heart disease. It also targets the poorest, people who are homeless, and those in prisons. It thrives in places where it is difficult if not impossible to implement the necessary social distancing, mask-wearing, and hand hygiene that can be the difference between life and death. It has precipitated the most severe global economic downturn seen in at least a century. Lockdowns in the poorest countries have had devastating consequences to lives and livelihoods, as Vinay Lal writes in his essay 'Viral Corona Capitalism'; and, as Chandrika Parmar adds in 'Swollen Feet', India's first lockdown led to the largest migration in the country's history when nearly 140 million newly unemployed people left the cities to return to towns and villages.

The deaths have not been evenly spread. More than half a million have been in the United States and the European Union, countries that are the world's biggest spenders on public health, and home to laboratories with some of the most advanced biomedical research facilities. In contrast, some of the lowest death rates are in the Asia-Pacific region, and in the countries of the Gulf, with the exception of Iran as Lila Randall notes in her article. As much of the world continued in the grip of second and third waves, life in China, New Zealand, Singapore, Thailand and Vietnam appeared to return to some kind of normal. And that includes economic and business life, too.

As with past pandemics in history, the coronavirus pandemic of 2020 will have longer-lasting effects. It will contribute to the changing balance of power between China and the United States; it will almost certainly contribute to lasting changes to how science is done and how medicines and vaccines are approved by regulatory bodies. It will affect how often we travel, how we travel and where we travel to. It likely will not impact the pace of industrialisation and urban development, but it will have other impacts that are as yet impossible to foresee.

I can remember sitting at my desk at the London offices of *Nature*, the primary journal of scientific research, overlooking King's Cross station. It was a few weeks after the first reports that an unknown virus had begun to filter out of Wuhan in China's Hubei province. This was late January 2020, and media were reporting some 300 cases. Although the overwhelming majority were in China, cases were beginning to be reported in Japan, South Korea and Thailand.

By January's third week, six people were known to have died, but we weren't completely sure whether the virus could transmit between humans. Even at that early stage, however, there were things we knew. Some of the first cases had been traced to a live animal market in Wuhan. The virus had also been identified as being in the same family of viruses that had caused Severe Acute Respiratory Syndrome (SARS) in the countries of East Asia, which had killed hundreds of people between 2002 and 2003. The SARS viruses infect humans via bats, a hardy animal with an extraordinary propensity to live with diseases, and the new coronavirus would subsequently be called SARS-CoV-2; and Covid-19 would be the name given to the disease.

As Colin Tudge points out, viruses are integral to ecosystems. Those that transmit diseases from animals to humans have been with us since the earliest times, and for as long as our two species have lived in shared spaces. But what are called zoonotic diseases seem to become more dangerous to humans, as humans continue to take over and convert natural habitats to serve human needs. HIV, which likely jumped to humans from chimpanzees, has infected around 75 million people and around 30 million people have died. The first SARS virus killed 15% of those infected, and half of those who were over sixty. In those first few days, I remember how tempting it was to think that the new coronavirus would be less lethal – only that assessment was fast changing.

Around the middle of January, researchers from a laboratory at Imperial College in London did some rapid modelling of people going in and out of Wuhan. On that basis, they estimated that there were at least 1,700 infections, and not 300. Looking at it now, it seems a trivial figure compared to what has happened since (nearly 90 million infections). But 1,700 was nearly six-times the number of reported cases, and to the untrained eye (in other words, most of us), that was a large multiple. Worse was to come as within days, China was preparing for the annual new year Spring Festival. If the Imperial College team was right, that meant the virus would potentially infect many more as hundreds of millions were planning on taking to the roads, rail and air, fanning out to all corners of China.

By common consent, the countries of the Asia-Pacific region have had much more success in taming the virus over the past twelve months, compared with the rest of the world. On my visits to China before the pandemic, I would often wonder why masks were commonly worn in public places – not only outdoors, to protect against pollution, but indoors in offices and in shopping centres, too. Clearly, they had absorbed the lessons from SARS. But there's one aspect that will forever be debated: should China – indeed, could China – have locked down in the final week of January 2020 and stopped people from travelling for the Spring Festival holidays. And if it had, what would the impact have been on the rest of the world? It's a question on which many papers will be written.

Critical questions are also being asked of the World Health Organization, which, by its own account, swung into action as quickly as it could. At the end of January, the WHO declared the virus to be a Public Health Emergency of International Concern. This is an official designation that is meant to trigger a cascade of actions by the world's public health agencies. In line with these actions, the WHO reminded all nations that they needed to test and isolate infected cases, and to do the same for the contacts of infected people. With the virus infecting people minute-by-minute, speed is of the essence. The WHO does not recommend creating some great technological infrastructure, but advises public authorities to recruit, train and deploy groups of community-health volunteers, locally-based, prepared to go house-to-house, door-to-door, checking on the health of households, identifying infected people, ensuring they stay home for a week or two, and then doing the same for their contacts. Pandemic management is a centuries-old practice as two essays in this issue from Nomanul Haq and Usama Hasan reveal. Our present knowledge has since been honed by the WHO after decades of experience working with health agencies tackling infectious diseases in the Global South.

Whereas countries in the Global South did indeed follow WHO advice, it was a different story in the northern hemisphere where the response continues to be inconsistent, contradictory, and which has cost lives. In the United States, the former president Donald J. Trump downplayed the virus's propensity to kill, disputed expert advice on social distancing and the wearing of masks, withheld support from states, and took the unconscionable decision to remove the nation's public health agency – the Centers for Disease Control and Prevention – from the heart of coronavirus decision-making. Policymakers in the US – and in many countries of the European Union – seem to have accepted that the virus should be allowed to circulate at a certain level, in line with how seasonal influenza is managed. What this action amounted to, in effect, was to tolerate a minimum level of what the actuarial and statistical communities call 'excess deaths'. Michael Rosen put it much more directly in his poem, *J'accuse*. 'J'accuse a small group of scientists of peddling the idea of "herd immunity" without vaccination as a viable and ethical policy even though they knew that it necessitated the deaths of hundreds of thousands of people,' he would write.

This was in contrast to the approach adopted by many leaders of Asia-Pacific countries, which sought to eliminate the virus altogether, aiming to have zero deaths on the grounds that every life is worth saving. But the leaders of the countries of the North did worse things than ignore WHO advice in those crucial early months.

Pandemics can bring out both the best and the worst in people and their governments. Cooperation and concern goes hand in hand with rule-breaking, corruption, competitive behaviour, and xenophobia. Reducing the risks of the latter is the key reason why viruses need to carry technical-sounding names, such as Sars-CoV-2, or HIV, and why they absolutely must not be named after identifiable people or places, according to an international agreement reached some years ago. But fate would mean that this pandemic arrived in the midst of an escalating trade war between China and the United States. China was becoming sensitive to criticisms that it could have acted faster, and its government officials are now starting to deny that it originated in Wuhan. For Trump, the Wuhan origins of the first cases, and that the WHO's director-general Tedros Adhanom Gebreyesus had close ties to China's leadership, gave enough reasons to call it the 'China virus', and accuse the WHO of being in China's pocket. Trump would eventually pull the plug on US membership of a global body that Washington had helped to bring to life seventy years ago.

The WHO often gets a bad rap during infectious disease outbreaks. Some expect the WHO to behave like the world's health service, which it cannot be on a budget which is far lower than what one developed country will spend on its public health in a year. Others criticise the agency for what in the past they have seen as undue alarmism. But the WHO works through a consensus of its member states, guided by researchers and public health bodies. It is far from perfect, but is unusual in the UN system in that expertise is more likely to trump other considerations in the search for best practice on what to do when there is a risk of harm, such as when an outbreak happens. Its advice is closely followed in countries that lack public health infrastructure. And when the coronavirus hit, countries in the Global South especially knew what they needed to do and got on with doing it. That seemed a bridge too far for Trump, and in his vindictiveness he moved to punish the agency for doing its job.

The rest of the world had more sense and stood firm against Trump's action, but pandemic nationalism takes many forms. Once a pandemic had been declared, nations needed to have sat down with each other and their science advisers, and try to come to a common understanding on some basic measures: for example, when to open and close borders; when to start and end lockdowns, and crucially, how to distribute vaccines once it became clear that these would be ready much earlier than expected. Such cooperation is equivalent to the first law in how to end a crisis in an interconnected system, as no country can be safe until every country is safe. It is how nations reacted when the 2008 Global Financial Crisis hit – ministers of finance quickly mobilised to recapitalise the banks. A different administration in the White House would almost certainly have coordinated a global pandemic response, but instead the past year has often been an object lesson in selfishness.

There is no greater example of this than in how vaccines will be distributed. The world has finite vaccine manufacturing capability and the vaccines now being authorised will need to be taken in two doses – a main dose and a booster, a few weeks apart. In a world of better channels to international cooperation, a system would be found to ensure some degree of equitable distribution. But at the time of writing, Australia, Canada, the United States and the United Kingdom had each pre-ordered between six and eight doses for each member of their populations. The European Union has pre-ordered nearly four doses for every person in their twenty-seven member states. The peoples of the Gulf states and the larger equatorial countries (Brazil, Mexico, India) are on track to receive two each. That still leaves something like 150 countries, including most of the continent of Africa, with little to no prospect of universal vaccine coverage during 2021.

In contrast to the actions of those we elect to lead us, the pandemic has had a different effect in the world of science. Researchers can easily match politicians and business people in a contest of ruthlessness and competitive behaviour. But the pandemic has also enabled many to show what science can achieve when researchers set aside the desire to compete and work towards a greater, shared goal. The speed of cooperation in science during this past year has been on a scale that I have not seen in more than twenty-five years in science journalism.

Credit here needs to go to China's researchers. Within days of those first cases of the virus, they were able to identify its unique genetic code. For decades, China's researchers have been collaborating with peers all over the world, so it was a no-brainer to see them upload this data to international databases for their peers around the world to access. These early actions enabled public health bodies in every country to develop coronavirus testing kits. And they allowed teams of researchers from different countries in a branch of science called structural biology to take this genetic information and use it to construct an image of what the virus looked like – the now famous spherical organism covered with spikes. This, too, was shared freely with the world, and enabled pharmaceutical companies, within days, to begin the task of designing vaccine candidates. That these candidates were being deployed just twelve months later is because regulatory bodies agreed to change their processes. Vaccines need to be tested on cells outside the human body, on different groups of human volunteers in a sequential process where one set of results often builds on the next. Some regulatory bodies allowed some of these processes to take place in parallel and encouraged pharmaceutical companies to provide them with access to data in real time (as opposed to at the end of trials).

The research underpinning all of this – from the biology of the virus, how it infects people, and how vaccines provide protection – still needed to be published in peer-reviewed journals to maintain confidence that short cuts were not taking place. But journals, too, changed their processes, in effect working around the clock across time-zones to assess the research coming their way. All of the world's research publishers ensured that all coronavirus research papers, past, present and future, would be free to access.

This was happening at the same time that researchers were themselves uploading and sharing their data and findings to websites known as 'preprints'. Conversation and critique are at the heart of the research process, but the pandemic had closed down many of the usual avenues where these conversations happen, especially scientific conferences. With many labs also shuttered, researchers turned to preprints to tell the world, and their peers, what they were doing – and in the process allowed hundreds, if not thousands more people, lay and expert, to become part of the research process. This is a development that will likely survive the pandemic, even as conferences and face-to-face working resumes.

It's not only preprints that are changing how science is communicated. The flow of scientific information has relied also heavily on social media. Twitter especially has been critical in conveying ideas; challenging new findings, or just alerting people to the existence of new research. This ability to communicate more quickly and more easily with vast numbers of people has a well-known downside, too. It is also fuelling what the

WHO has been calling an 'infodemic' – a pandemic of misinformation and 'disinformation' – misinformation that is deliberately aimed at misleading. As Nidhal Guessoum shows, none of this is new, but social media has inserted rocket boosters underneath fringe ideas, allowing them to penetrate vastly more numbers of people than would have been possible in the past.

Social media is especially fuelling vaccine hesitancy, though, paradoxically, people with vaccine-sceptical views are now more likely to be found in the developed countries. People in countries with few pre-pandemic memories of what it means to battle an infectious disease seem to have become complacent about the value of vaccination, and why it is essential to protecting against disease. So, although their governments have gone ahead and pre-ordered the overwhelming majority of the world's vaccine stock, it is not yet clear whether sufficient numbers will agree to take the jab for their nations to be fully protected against contracting the Covid-19 disease.

The rapid development of vaccines has shown what collaboration can achieve. Indeed, the world possesses the means to defeat the pandemic within a year. It will take an enormous effort, a combination of leadership and logistics, but sufficient vaccines could be distributed to vaccinate the world if there is a will to do this. As Anwar Ibrahim writes so movingly on his experiences with institutions of politics and democracy, 'the notion of justice has been mythologised through a great many historical impediments. Casting it as some higher form, forgetting that it is lived tradition, it becomes a peak we can no longer summit'. Having so comprehensively mismanaged the pandemic, justice demands that the leaders of the developed nations, those with the means to produce and buy vaccines, now take steps towards equitable vaccine distribution. Sufficient vaccines will soon exist for all of the world's peoples to be vaccinated. In my fleeting moments of optimism, I believe it could happen. Even if it is a summit, it is one we can climb!

JUSTICE FOR A PRAYING PERSON

Anwar Ibrahim

Human beings require movement. Just as we reach the end of one motion, we have already started planning the next. If we are stopped, we figure out a way to go again. If we truly must be still, then we need to socialise, which is, in and of itself, movement of another type. And even when we are at our most powerless in provoking ourselves onward, that most beautiful organ, the human brain picks up the pace for the sake of progress. Immovability is an existential crisis. Our ontologies are quickly made inadequate before reality and the uncomfortable chill of panic looms heavy. This has been a refreshed, but definitely not a refreshing, experience for us recently as a consequence of the coronavirus. A lesson we can all take from our collective trauma under the Covid-19 global pandemic. We keep repeating the line that 'we are all in this together,' but can we look away from the mirror? This discomfort we all feel must couple with various headlines and platitudes that are all pointing to, and rather verbosely, the fact that things are not right. There have been indicators along the way and we have all picked up on them in one way or another. But we paid only slight attention to them and allowed them to be normalised. The grinding halt of the world before the virus gave us the whiplash that primes an individual for learning, but our inability to put a face on the problem gives power to our devices of normalisation. After all time keeps moving and so ought we.

The clock keeps ticking and the present carries on. The virus shines a light on many trends established prior to the pandemic – racism endemic to societies all around the world, existential fears that drive dehumanising identity politics or hateful xenophobia, and the horrific inequalities our global economic systems readily perpetuate. Anyone who is different or foreign was libelled to bring this disease into our homes. Chinese and Asians around the world found themselves again on the receiving end of a familiar tune. Muslims around the world were targeted by wayward conspiracy theories which, of course, is not a new phenomenon. But because a mosque gathering turned into a super spreader event, it has to be rationalised that all mosques everywhere were hives of infectivity. There are no clear statistics for the number of migrant workers who have been victims, both directly and indirectly to the disease since most countries don't count them as actual people. Therefore, it is deemed acceptable to pay them less and stick them in accommodations we barely deem tolerable for prisoners. Close confinement, poor sanitation and without the PPE to spare beyond those who can afford it. What did we expect, that our lack of acknowledgement would keep them safe? The United States demonstrated nicely how withholding acknowledgement of reality works out in the end. And suffering with the migrant worker, abandoned to die far from home, are the poor, who never had a chance from the start, abandoned to die without a home in their homelands. While millions joined the ranks of the unemployed and impoverished, those already below our dramatically underestimated poverty lines, sunk deeper into pre-existing inequalities without anything to grab onto and maybe pull themselves back up with. The circumstances left available to the global poor only made them prime targets on the pandemic's warpath.

SARS-CoV-2, the virus that causes the disease known as Covid-19, is said to be particularly severe for those suffering from 'underlying conditions'. These are such things as cardiac problems, diabetes, and cancers. In the early days of the pandemic, this was used by some to argue that those with underlying conditions had it coming anyway, so it is unfair to stop the rest of us from going shopping and getting on with our busy social lives. Of course, all of us suffer from an underlying condition of being mortal. But there is another underlying condition I want to focus on: justice, or rather its conspicuous and almost universal absence.

Even before the pandemic, I was in lockdown: three times, confined to the four walls of a prison cell. Little compares to the immobilisation imposed by a prison sentence, particularly one uplifted by bogus charges. Regardless of the manoeuvring that saw to me finding myself behind those bars, the terror came in the denial of movement. Even the manufactured images of movement pandered by hollow, dead yards and echoing halls held little weight and the bliss of ignorance faded quickly. I did manage one comfort and escape. The one permitted through books. Eventually I could gallivant off in one of the masterful works of Shakespeare or engross myself in a challenging and stimulating intellectual work, a dream of a better tomorrow. But I was a political prisoner and anything deemed subversive was strictly forbidden. So, Hamlet and political philosophy would have to bide their time. I was, at least, allowed a copy of the Holy Qur'an. Since nothing in there ever led anyone towards any radical ideas about how to change a society. Aside from my prison Qur'an, I had one other book at my disposal. It was given to me by a colleague with the note that this ought to be where I focus my intellectual energies and learn the error of my ways. It was a book of prayer.

This particular book of prayer was *Munyatul Musalli*, written by the nineteenth century Malay scholar Shaykh Daud bin Abdullah Al-Fatani. *Munyatul Musalli* translates from Arabic as 'the dream of a praying person', and is perhaps familiar to Muslim students in the Middle East and South East Asia. It is a detailed instruction guide that notes the various prayers and rituals associated with them. Rather elementary, but beggars are rarely granted the freedom to be choosers. I took to Al-Fatani, bounding for the motion guaranteed in recounting all the prayers, their etiquette, and even a step-by-step playbook for the *hajj*. Reading through the disciplined articulations, I was suddenly struck when I happened upon the final chapter. Seeming a bit out of place, it was a discussion of justice, and it definitely had my attention. What did a philosophical discussion of justice have to do with a practical manual to prayer?

Although this sudden change of tone was not all that out of the ordinary. Rather, it adhered to a fairly common practice where a scholarly discussion would be nightcapped with a *tatmimul faedah*, or concluding benefit. Like an epilogue, but more of an author's note, the last words amplified the text beyond the page. This practice, in accordance with the *Shari'ah*, would apply the discussion at hand to the day-to-day business of the intended audience. The original audience intended for *Munyatul Musalli* was the Sultan (which one remains a topic of debate) who commissioned the work. Al-Fatani saw fit that his additional benefit be a chapter of anecdotes on how a ruler might improve the overall wellbeing of his society by practicing just governance. This anecdotal presentation of justice spoke to a greater pan-Asian practice that was commonly used throughout the

Malay Archipelago. It is also the method of teaching favoured by the Chinese masters Confucius and Sun-Tzu for their students and advising Emperors or civil servants.

One such anecdotal vignette notes how ancient rulers used to give their ministers three pages which contained messages that are to be given to the ruler when their reign tipped towards tyranny or wrath. The pages remind the ruler, first, that they are not God and shall return to the dust, second, that demonstrating mercy on Earth will ensure its reflection in the Hereafter, and third, that the ruler's duty to uphold justice in accordance with Allah's law has no compensation. Another series of anecdotes features a farm animal or agricultural product that yields surplus but when stolen by the ruler only yields deficit as the maintenance of justice was the cause of the originally yielded surplus, thus only when the magical source of wealth is returned to the people that justice is reinstated. Other anecdotes speak to the quality of the ruler's advisors. It compares viziers to the gates of a city or as a mirror of the ruler themselves. If they do not reflect the values of the ruler, then the blemishes also present on the rulers. The general idea of justice crafted by these stories is one in which respect is paid to a proper order in society, especially concerning distribution of wealth and goods. The justice spoken of here was installed by God, but requires practical and ongoing refinement by all humanity, rulers and the ruled. Subtly, the responsibility incumbent on participants in a just society is alluded to along with justice being an ongoing process as opposed to the Western notion of it being a heavenly idea to be aspired to.

One could read Al-Fatani's final thought as his chance to take advantage of his position. Perhaps, in preparing a guide for the Sultan to perform hajj with a local's fluidity, he could sneak in a few of his own political opinions in that clever way intellectuals like to do with their words. I disagree with this assessment. I feel Al-Fatani was aiming at a much more profound end. As I pored over the book of prayer I fell into deep reflection. Prayer is an institution that is fundamentally central to being a Malay. One could make this claim about any community in touch with its religious identity, but for Malays and the rest of the Ummah where Arabic is not our first language, and our culture diverges greatly from our brothers and sisters in the Middle East, our adherence and respect for prayer makes for a point of strong connection between Malays and the Ummah. In this steeped tradition of prayer, we also find a deep commitment to justice. Al-Fatani not only teases at an entangled relationship between prayer and justice, he highlighted the direct role each of them plays within the hearts and acts of Muslims, being an integral, deeply embedded part of Muslim tradition. Coming at it from the Christian tradition, I think to the American philosopher Cornell West, who famously noted in his book, *Race Matters*, that 'justice is what love looks like in public.' In Islam, we continue this sentiment; justice is what prayer looks like in public. In exploring this idea, we must elevate justice beyond its current buzz word status so that it may live and breathe again in a world that has allowed it to go too long neglected into atrophy.

While there have been a few good ideas here and there, the Western pursuit of justice in many aspects has been a categorical failure. Sure, justice has occasionally been allowed to shine when convenient, for the privileged few, but 'justice for all', well, this is fantastical delusion. And it would be fair to ask, then why we should run the gambit from Hobbes to Rawls, as I intend to do? What have they actually done for the West, never mind the rest? The answer to this question is multifaceted. Some elements of Western control, due to its dominance over the last couple of centuries, go deeper than formal rule. The power to define has not only kept the West in its dominance through the supremacy of language and thought, it has also established a set of norms which cannot simply be cast away, but need to be transcended. For true transformative change to take place, a change that could even overturn the era of Western dominance, the successes and failures of the West ought to be taken note of, built upon, and criticised. The alternative would be a foolish pursuit of a new way that ignores history, the complexity of the modern world, and rides dangerously close to narcissism. So, we learn Western political theory and analyse Shakespeare not just because they are enjoyable, or because this is what the former British overlords decreed, or even because it is the end all, be all of enlightened thinking, but because it is there and we can learn from it. And how would we be any better than the colonisers if we took an entire worldview, tag it as treachery, and tried to set about reinventing the wheel, doomed on multiple fronts to repeat the same tragedies and comedies? And in postnormal times, it is about polylogue, which requires as many different voices and viewpoints, even if they have a history of violence against us and even if they are blatantly wrong. If we can see what's wrong, perhaps we might be persuaded to do right. And from within, using the voices of those who have held power in the past, we can bring in our own voices and the voices of others. It is slow, it is an exhausting struggle, but short of brutality or the risk of greater injustice, it is the only way to go about lasting change. Granted, a lot of barricades require tearing down first, particularly for Muslim thought.

The notion of justice has been mythologised through a great many historical impediments. Casting it as some higher form, forgetting that it is lived tradition, it becomes a peak we can no longer summit. Despite justice being embedded in Islamic scholarship, and being a fundamental objective of its adherents, we do not talk about it. Injustice is taken as given and we have almost surrendered our agency over justice in the real world. Modernity consigned justice to a nebulous notion of egalitarianism. Its basic aim was to keep the wheels of production turning to ensure constant growth, perpetual progress, and assume that some benefits would trickle down to the down trodden. Postmodernism does us no better. The discussion devolved into 'justice for whom' or 'justice with respect to what'. The holistic totality of justice thrown to the wind. Objective justice has been assassinated. In this subjectivity, we reduce justice to a notion of exchange. As if it could be a commodity anyone would want to trade on the floor of the stock exchange. Left unspoken it becomes quieter than a whisper, a noise at the mercy of a cacophony of background sounds.

That noise crescendos into focus with the wrapping of a gavel. The sound that brings an auction to order, that once punctuated my school house debates, should have easily evolved into the thumping that filled the void between our arguments on the floor of Malaysia's Parliament. Instead, this romantic flow of musical notes was interrupted by the collisions which set the tempo for my appearances in the courtroom. The noise at the collision between gavel and sound block is hardly distinguishable from the impact of the policeman's baton against my body. In the 1970s, during my rebellious university days, a courtroom wasn't always necessary. That colonial vestige, the Internal Securities Act (ISA), made it so that formal charges were not required to detain me or anyone else deemed an enemy of the state. As I grew older, I would at least be upgraded to farcical show-trial. A matinee sure to ruin anyone's afternoon.

During my various detentions, I learned there is a certain naivety amongst revolutionaries. You learn that the limits of injustice are not simply wrongful imprisonment or tyrannical despots, injustice is far more clever and more so often less obvious. There is a tendency to confine justice to the business of robed lawyers and armchair philosophers, but it is rather curious how it is the hot topic of those pitted against the threat of imprisonment and those who find themselves behind bars. When one is the victim of wrong doing, there is a desire to seek pity from the mirror, but mirrors are few and far between in these cells. There is no choice but to face reality. My condition was not new, nor was I alone. I now shared in a history common to many held in Malaysia or other former colonies throughout the world. Victims of laws created to divide a collected people and control them. And that history lived on the faces of my fellow inmates. I learned all too well the truth behind the American writer Mark Twain's quote 'if you want to see the dregs of society, go down to the jail and watch the changing of the guard.' And when you realise where these people with whom I now shared a place had come from, you understand that what happens here is just a microcosm for what is happening out there each and every day. I can count my blessings as at least out there I could move, yet in or out, many of my fellow inmates never even had a chance at motion. For the disadvantaged and impoverished, their imprisonment began at birth and would extend far beyond the most corrupt courts' decree.

On their faces were written the contemporary problem of justice. And the problem at hand goes much deeper than what is often credited. The faces behind injustice, or more appropriately the absence of justice, invoke the reality, which we would rather ignore, behind poverty and those pushed away as outliers of society. And in our ignorance, we deny them the dignity we thought was inalienable to human beings. Even in prison, where one might think at least there is the mutual impediment on one's freedoms to unite us, the inequalities outside the prison gates are as much, and perhaps more so, made apparent. Today, as the Covid-19 pandemic runs on, we exhaust the safety nets we had, which were generally not even prepared to handle the first wave of shutdowns the virus demanded. The fragility of our comfort and security in these uncertain times echoes a turning of the screw on injustices around the world.

The Shakespeare I once thought of as a mode of escape, told familiar tales that ring too real. 'For as thou urgest justice, be assured Thou shall have justice, more than thou desir'st.' I had desired perhaps Portia's monologue in appeal to mercy, yet this line from *The Merchant of Venice* is indicative of the togetherness we all too often forget pertains to justice. The seventeenth century English poet, John Donne penned a similar meditation which would go on to inspire Ernest Hemingway's novel *For Whom the Bell Tolls*.

> No man is an island, entire of itself; every man is a piece of the continent, a part of the main. If a clod be washed away by the sea, Europe is the less, as well as if a promontory were, as well as if a manor of thy friend's or of thine own were: any man's death diminishes me, because I am involved in mankind, and therefore never send to know for whom the bell tolls; it tolls for thee.

Donne's bells are that of the churches in England which rang either to signal a wedding or a funeral. These tolls were for the latter. Yet, he might well have spoken of the popular retributive characteristic of modern justice. But let us not forget Mahatma Gandhi's quote about an eye for an eye. As humans we are all united in various commonalities, especially our own mortality. One individual's death then is not just a loss for the individual or those close to them, but a loss for us all. A loss for our community. A loss for the great human journey. Or, as to put it in the terms of the Qur'an, 'if anyone kills a person…it is as he kills all mankind' (5:32). This lesson bears a great weight in these unprecedented times when all of us are at the mercy of Covid-19. Hemingway provides us with an interesting example. In his novel, he takes note that Spain's trading of democracy for fascism and dictatorship which followed the Spanish Civil War, was not just a loss for Spain, but for the international community and the beautiful idea of democracy. It was a stain on the progress promised after the atrocities of the twentieth century. Somewhere along the line justice lost its living, breathing quality, doomed to fossilisation.

This resultant ossification is a problem of mentality. The corresponding manufactured interregnum on justice discourse is not just a fault of culture, but the very structural pedestal upon which the West confined justice. It has been made into a sort of perfection, an ideal state, that can never be achieved. And who wants to be Sisyphus? This is the origin of the academic taking-for-granted-of the concept of justice. Students learn of Plato's ideal city or Aristotle's virtuous man. Ethics and just actions are then confined to the inaccurate calculous of the middle way. It is a tragic interpretation of the famous line from the American author John Steinbeck's *East of Eden*. 'And now that you don't have to be perfect, you can be good.' Originally this line was meant to combat the modernist craving to be perfect at the expense of morality, but when taken in consideration of the history of Western discourse on justice, it appears to be the rejection of perfection so as to deny the responsibility of morality. If you can't be good, at least you tried. This mentality carried on in the development of Christendom and the state in the West. Today it infects the academic industrial complex of Western disciplines from Perth to Paris and Timbuktu to Kuala Lumpur and beyond. This intellectual block is very difficult to break through. Guilty of this myself, we often say, we need to be more critical in our thinking or provoke greater creativity and imagination. But to what end? How do we do this? Are we not confounded upon launch? How does the West out think itself? And perhaps for too long we have waited for this sort of revelation to be delivered from on high, instead of seeking it out.

There was a moment of hope in the West with the arrival of the Enlightenment. Such a storm of turmoil ought to have shaken a few things up. The state, the church, the arts, and humanity's place among it all was brought into question. Following the Classic period, most conceptual discussions were restricted to looking for biblical justifications for the truth claims made by the pagans of yesteryear, or to letting them be damned to eternal hellfire. Their diligent work gave the framework by which Latin America has been burning since the colonial period and such abominations as just-war theory. The Enlightenment called for new ideas, needed to fill in the gaps left by Christianity and feudal society. This also kicked off the great secularisation of Europe which claims to be riding strong in the sophistication of the European Union today. And most pertinent for our discussion here, justice was put on trial.

But one does not simply remove justice from the pedestal the ancient Greeks put it upon. To do so would tarnish the concept, making it somewhat less. So, a vessel must be created to keep intact the perfect nature of justice. The Enlightenment thinkers devised the *social contract* to do just that and to build up to what we must go back to, the *state of nature*. An obvious allusion to the Garden of Eden, it is the port of call for the journey to be taken towards perfect justice – anchored on freedom, a notion that has become the pride and nightmare of Western civilisation. For thinkers of the Enlightenment, freedom is unbridled. Freedom at the cost of all else, including responsibility, or the survival concerns of society. This is a major divergence from the notion of freedom in Islam and other non-Western thought. This was freedom from structure, shame, order, and, where natural law dictated, the way of the world. Humans – and bear in mind the definition of such a creature was rather exclusive at this point in history – endowed with reason would exit the state of nature by way of the social contract, conquering everything – and apparently everyone – along the way. The total freedom of the state of nature had to be sacrificed or negotiated with an ordering entity dubbed the *sovereign*. Thoughts range the spectrum from absolute rulers to true rule by all. Monarchy, dictatorship, oligarchy, republic, and democracy were given a long overdue critical analysis. For Thomas Hobbes, the state of nature was a dangerous dog-eat-dog world and a citizen must surrender all their freedoms to their sovereign, a powerful absolute tyrant, the titular character of his 1651 opus, *Leviathan*. John Locke took more stock in these freedoms or rights, seeing them as sacred and inalienable. The point of the social contract was to check the sovereign, who he thought ought to be rather a body composed of the people, whose purpose is to defend the rights which pertain to a citizen's preservation of 'life, liberty, and property'. Jean-Jacques Rousseau was more of a democracy extremist. His idea of the state of nature was more puritanical than Hobbes and the structures of society have robbed humanity of its ability to be truly free. The social contract thus was instituted to emulate the freedom of the state of nature without disrupting the practicality of history. Equality, liberty, and fraternity were of the greatest rights that small, localised democracies must actively engage with to perfect. These men stand out in an age of rigorous debate and ripe ideas of how to build a better world, at least for some.

The idealist sentiment of justice continued to look at society in a vacuum, as a subject in the lab. Society rarely ever survives under such conditions. A theory was needed to allow for practical progress that did not diminish the perfection of justice. Enter Jeremy Bentham and John

Stewart Mill. Given such an imperfect world, there must be a simple categorisation which can provide for a ready-to-hand calculous. While the outcome may not always be perfect, we are only human, and the hope is it will come as close as possible. This is the rationality behind utilitarianism. The world was thus simplified into pains and pleasures, and the objective of society was to bring about the most pleasure for the greatest amount. Obviously, in our imperfect world, we cannot please everyone, but we will try. And so, the trap that created the manufactured justice discourse interregnum was revved up for another go. Here we hear the echoes of Winston Churchill, his words spoken on Armistice Day of 1947 that sum up the accomplishment of a history of Western notions of justice.

> Many forms of Government have been tried, and will be tried in this world of sin and woe. No one pretends that democracy is perfect or all-wise. Indeed, it has been said that democracy is the worst form of Government except for all those other forms that have been tried from time to time.

You can see the hopelessness in such a mentality? Yet this excerpt is quoted as though it were a national anthem. What motivation is there for innovation and progress where perfection is the impossible and yet the goal? This great contradiction in Western thought ushered in an era of catastrophic failures and lessons left unlearned, not just for the West, but for the world the West colonised. Its colonial power was strongest not only in the land it controlled via labyrinthine administrations or divide and conquer policy, but also in the toxic education they felt burdened with imparting on those they called 'savages'. Us, who had to fight for the simple recognition as humans with the capacity for reason and thus worthy of citizenship. It is no wonder the postmodern thinkers thrived so much on the husks of hollow morality and brittle ethics. Not dissimilar to Dante's descent into hell, perhaps a fitting disclaimer should be placed upon the history of justice in Western thought. 'Abandon all hope, ye who enter here.'

American philosopher John Rawls aimed to provide some hope when in 1971 he published *A Theory of Justice*. Rawls primarily wanted to give a contemporary defence of social contract theory using the hot new method of the time, analytic philosophy. He needed to put to rest the popularity and ease with which utilitarianism and right-wing libertarianism was sweeping across much of Western political thought once and for all. Gaia weeps that such a wave of thought could not be curbed. Presumably, in Rawls's mind, he had accomplished the objectives he set out for, yet its ending was less than satisfying. In reopening the pandora's box on justice, one expects more resolution for the ills of the times, so it goes, many of which persist today.

Rawls transformed the discourse on justice from looking for the ideal world to something more practical. He decided that what we needed to do first is to derive the important principles that make a just society. It was to be the *veil of ignorance,* which would ensure fairness above all and also break down social inequalities and tyrannical structures. To determine the principles of a just society, each member would enter *the original position*, which sounds like the state of nature, but is more like a very plain conference room used for a market research study. Wealth, class, family, birthplace, citizenship status, employment and so on would all be left to the realm of the unknown for participants in the original position under the veil of ignorance. In the parlance of postnormal times, this would be second order or 'vincible' ignorance. You are aware that these categories exist, but you do not know which one the lottery of life will draw for you. In this position, the participants are forced to find principles that benefit the worst off in a given society, lest it be you for whom the bell tolls! This set up allows for two major tenants of *justice as fairness* to arise. First, each person in a given society will have equal rights and access to the most basic fundamental liberties. Second, if there must be inequalities, then the only allowable ones are those that benefit the worst off in society. In accordance with the first principle, the benefits of these inequalities must be open and equally available to all members of society.

The publication of *A Theory of Justice* stirred the sleeping giant of Western political philosophy. Fifty years on, Rawls is making a comeback after Donald Trump's divisive presidency forced the American liberals to confront the issues of injustice, inequality and social division all over again. Ironically, Rawls and his greatest academic nemesis, Robert Nozick, held offices in the same department at Harvard University. Nozick leaned towards a rights-based approach that would rally the libertarians who stood against Rawls's liberal dreamland. Rawls garnered criticism from friend, foe, and many non-Western scholars and thinkers. How does justice as fairness account for the dynamics of the family unit, for women's rights, or the inherent injustice in the capitalist system? Others questioned his reliance on structures. He believed that institutions devised under the veil of ignorance could do no wrong. This, of course, was a major attacking point for Nozick who held to a minimalist state. For him, the structures Rawls hoped to pin victory on, would be the noose that hanged people's fundamental rights. Nozick leaves notions of charity and social justice outside the jurisdiction of the state. After all, he claims, abiding by the script of Austrian-British economist, Friedrich Hayek, that we could not possibly know what is truly needed by every citizen to establish a truly equitable society. Thus, we should not rob the rights of one for the benefit of the other in the hope that the maths works out in the end. The Rawls-Nozick divide is a major segment of the line upon which Republicans and Democrats in the US debate. Both agreed that justice must be derived from principles. Yet both men fell into familiar pitfalls. They had each developed a utopian system, and people needed practical, real-world solutions to the impending doom of inequality that kept on creeping as we approached the last chapter of the twentieth century. The problem seemed, again, that Western scholars could not out think the West they found themselves within.

An Indian economist and Nobel laureate would provide an answer to the major failures of Rawls's theory, particularly to non-Western cultures; and he would do this in a way that would not completely dismiss the theory, rather adapt, adjust and take it further. Amartya Sen's work *The Idea of Justice*, dedicated to Rawls himself, would not only bring a non-Western voice to the discourse on justice, but seek to build a bridge so that a more plural approach could make the way for a more just world. Sen defends Rawls's approach noting that it cannot be universalised. There are countless ways to get to justice and as long as one path does not itself involve the violation of justice, then logically it is a good path. Infused with anecdotes and Indian scripts, Sen not only opens the theory up to justice, he does it in the language and mentality of the West. The value of *The Idea of Justice* is that it speaks to a diverse, multilanguage, interdisciplinary approach to justice. 'What is presented here is a theory of justice in a very broad sense. Its aim is to clarify how we can proceed to address questions of enhancing justice and removing injustice, rather than to offer resolutions of questions about the nature of perfect justice', he writes. Finally, a theory that offers practicality for the Western pursuits of justice.

With the question, 'why should the status of intense economic needs, which can be matters of life and death, be lower than that of personal liberties?', Sen opens justice up to the realm of economics more specifically. A critical point as it is in economic injustice that we see some of the greatest suffering in our contemporary times. He emphasises that the earliest economic theoreticians held the preservation of justice as tantamount to a viable theory of economics. Similar to his stance on the multicultural necessity of a justice discourse, we can assume that Sen would approve of a transdisciplinary approach to seeking justice. Justice, especially in what we now consider postnormal times, must be a polylogue. Justice is multiplicity and need not be some supernatural entity which even Shakespeare leaves to the determination of higher beings, 'and let time try'. Rather, why do we not do something about it?

Yet before we can go further, we have run into a bi-polar impediment. Covid-19 is not the only viral entity that has seized up progress. On one side of this impediment, we see the Western pursuit of justice has reached an impasse of contradictions. The pursuit of justice, as ideal utopia or practical guidance, cannot reconcile with the competing Western interests of neoliberal capitalism and the ossified tradition-bound pseudo democracy the global standard hails as infallible. The slings and arrows suffered by the global poor are the background noise to the enabling of unmitigated inequalities and the normality that pervades the privileged individual's capacity to exist above the law. Indeed, the ghost of Westminster are felt in the farthest reaches of the former British Empire and the Western monopoly on definition extends without bounds, confounding even the Islamic attempt at a reasoned justice. On the other hand, this impediment is the diminishing of any intellectual pursuits by Muslim scholars. This is well illustrated in Khaled Abou El Fadl's *Reasoning with God*, where he has to spend an extended preface sanitising Islamic law, Muslim law, Shari'ah, and *fiqh* from the misinterpretations and false claims, made by both non-Muslims and Muslims alike, that have confounded these concepts before he can even try bringing them into the contemporary context. This dual-natured stalemate is not only ridiculous, it reveals why the discussion itself cannot get any traction in the contemporary world. The status-quo is allowed to flourish and run amok. And this is what we are so eager to get back to after the pandemic? I would hope not.

In contrast to Western scholars, Muslim thinkers of the classical period had two major advantages. First, it was not of great importance to these thinkers whether their sources were Muslim or not. Islam does not see itself as separate from history. Perhaps the biblical language of 'God's chosen people' established a major hurdle in separating the praiseworthy from heresy. The Qur'an clearly states that God's revelation to the Prophet Muhammad is for all humankind, believer or not, Arab or otherwise. This revelation is also the last in a series, thus prior scriptures or writings are there to be studied and for gaining knowledge and wisdom. After all, who can discredit the great advancements in thinking that came before the Qur'anic revelation, and for the thinkers of Muslim civilisations, what an opportunity it proved to build upon the past as they did in numerous fields of inquiry. Second, classical Muslim thinkers were not trapped in dualities and categories. This obsession of Western thinkers has bedevilled the minds of generations. The dichotomies of mind, body, soul, or what have you were not as rigidly abided in the Islamic thinking of the time as it was in the West. Islamic thought was more open to blending and working with synthesis, less concerned with the precise dissections and clear-cut demarcations of their Western contemporaries.

The early Christian Church rose to a position of power largely based on its liturgical structuring. The very relationship between believer and Creator, God, required the intermediary of the clergy, from a common priest to the highest intermediary, the Pope. This may have begun out of the need for a literate member of the community to read the message of the Bible, but this role quickly evolved into a lucrative source of power, reaching its apex with the selling of indulgences. The Church not only rose to hold power over who would and would not receive salvation, but political and territorial power also. Islam did not have this history as it did not have a clergy, even though some *ulama* – religious scholars – did hold a prestigious position in society. Maturing in a culture more attuned to the oral tradition and the Prophet himself being unlettered, the relationship between believer and God was more personal. This personal relationship required that humanity had a responsibility and stake in the world they lived in with the perks of freedom and the Hereafter. The competing or cooperating interests of church and state were thus not as contentious. As both the Western and Islamic civilisations continued to do as humans do and spread across the map, they were bound to meet, or in the words of Samuel Huntington, clash.

As the West rose to dominance, so did its views, histories, and internal problems for everyone under its influence. By way of analogy, the failures of the early Christian Church were thrust upon Islam. And somewhere in history a rumour started that Islam will not get you to the truth, as it is just a religion – or to others, a heresy – and because of this it cannot come about the creation of something so pure and secular as democracy. And now a common belief holds that Islam cannot get to where the West is unless it first undergoes its own Enlightenment or an equivalent. But I call the West's bluff. I look at their constitutions, and more importantly the debates that forged these great documents; what is not directly copied and pasted from scripture is hardly distinguishable from moral ethics derived from a worldview informed by the Christian faith and ethical framing. And that doesn't have to be a problem. Many different framings can lead one to a logical conclusion of right from wrong. So why not Islam? And isn't it best to get as many reasons for what is right or what is wrong as possible. Is this not the scholar's errand and must it not be undertaken meticulously and with a critical lens? And after all, is this really what anyone wants? Who says Muslim societies wish to match the position of the West, failed stewards of the Earth confounded by their fundamentalist individualism and corruption rotted systems of distribution and justice? And what did the Enlightenment get Europe? Two world wars and a century of destruction and atrocity, upwards of one hundred million casualties, and destruction of Other cultures and traditions on a mass scale. 'The Enlightenment legacy', writes Ziauddin Sardar,

> that Islam and Europe have nothing in common, that Islam is only a darker shadow of the West, that liberal secularism is the destiny of all human cultures, is much in evidence in our newspapers and television, literature and scholarship, as well as in our politics and foreign policies. It is the bedrock of Francis Fukuyama's 'End of History' hypothesis, Samuel Huntington's 'Clash of Civilization' thesis, and the neo-conservative 'Project for the New American Century'. *Voltaire's Bastards*, to use the title of John Ralston Saul's brilliant 1992 book, are busy rationalising torture, military interventions, western supremacy

> and demonising Islam and Muslims. The Enlightenment may have been big on reason but it was, as Saul shows so convincingly, bereft of both meaning and morality. Forgive me if I don't stand up and salute the Enlightenment.

We need to get over the notion that the West has won history and, therefore, the right to tell the story of the past for all and set the terms for the future of everyone. The rule that anything and everything must be done for the maintenance of supremacy of the West needs to end. And despite the reams of evidence to support this, perhaps the global cataclysm of Covid-19 will really open our eyes. There are other stories out there and other paths to reach the things we as humans stand united in desiring.

The Islamic discourse of the classical period was a global discourse. The history of Islam, as Marshall Hodgson shows in his multi-volume *The Venture of Islam*, was world history. Abu Nasr Al-Farabi, a tenth century Muslim philosopher, held Aristotle as the 'first teacher' and in accordance with this adoration, was known as the 'second teacher'. He delighted in as much Plato as he could get his hands on. He even wrote of how the Prophet Muhammad was the philosopher king Plato longed for in *Republic*. From the constitution of Medina to the construction of the State, the Prophet's examples demonstrate that a just society, as Plato and al-Farabi longed for, can be realised. This was not a lofty aspiration but a realistic goal that can be achieved. Ibn Rushd aligned with Al-Farabi's thinking, emphasising the critical role philosophy plays in political order and justice. Just as the Prophet lived the philosophical ideal, it is incumbent on all humans to follow this example. The Qur'an asks us to be just, for Ibn Rushd, this is a call to philosophise. For critical thought and contemplation must take place for all politicians and law practitioners. Otherwise, we are just applying the law and this is insufficient for the fulfilment of the definition of justice. This is only a sample of the global discourse that extended from Baghdad to Andalusia with Ibn Bajja and Ibn-Tufayl.

Postcolonial spirit and revived Muslim nationalism between the 1970s and 1990s show that the Muslim intellectual exploration of justice followed a similar trajectory to the West. Many of their calls and intellectual efforts took the Western scaffolding as given and tried to Islamify or Shari'ahfy it. Opponents to this approach, such as Sardar and Merryl Wyn Davies point to how this makes the *Islamised* idea subservient to and subject to the same flaws as the Western paradigms. Islamic economics, taken from the approach of using the Shari'ah to justify neoliberal economics, not only makes it a sub-field of Economics, a Western discipline, but also subject to the same rampant inequalities and exploits as its overlord. The urgent project now is to move from 'Islamisation' to integration of knowledge.

To help in refuting the mischaracterisations of Shari'ah, Khaled Abou El Fadl's boils it down to its original definition so that you are not tempted to immediately make the jump to Islamic jurisprudence. Shari'ah, simply put, is a path to water. Water, being a pretty useful find in a desert climate, extrapolated, it is a pathway to nourishment or the good. The brilliance of El Fadl comes in his positioning of openness as fundamental to Islam. Islam is God's final message, but not his *only* message. Shari'ah could readily refer to the laws of Moses, the path of Jesus, or the tradition or life of the Prophet Muhammad. It is this openness that stood as the bedrock to *La Convivencia* of Umayyad Spain and will be the key to building a global Convivencia where people differing in culture, language, ethnicity, religion, and any other identity label may be able to live together. This is religion at its highest level, religion that expounds a universal perspective, religion that heals bigotry and fanaticism. This is not a call for uniformity, as if such a dream could practically be imposed. Look at the difficulty we have all seen in getting the public to follow the safety protocols for the pandemic when their lives truly depend on it. We need a global togetherness where we can simultaneously cherish difference and cherish our own identities.

This sentiment abounds in the work of Afghani legal scholar Mohammad Hashim Kamali. His writings on justice not only revive Islamic approaches to knowledge but demonstrate how it can be a standard of which the rest of the world ought to take notice. Kamali importantly separates justice, *adl*, from Shari'ah. The misconception is that the only way to attain justice is through Shari'ah. Kamali says that while Shari'ah ought always to be aimed at seeking justice or a just world, it is not necessarily the only way, 'since justice is an overriding objective, the quest towards it is not just confined to justice under the rule of law, but should be pursued at all levels, within or outside existing law.' This harkens back to Al-Fatani's notion of justice as the ultimate lived practice of prayer. Kamali maintains the openness seen in El Fadl, not only examining it beside other non-Muslim sources, but in locating it in the contemporary world. He interestingly places justice in a triumvirate of values with equality and freedom. One sacrificed for the others sees the strong triangle topple. Justice after all, as described in the Qur'an, is fundamentally a balance. And even this notion is not the advent of Islam, Islam did not appear out of nothingness, it came to a world where the clock had already been ticking in a region that was a crossroads to trade and cultures. The notion of justice as balance is also seen in the Vedic tradition of India and is played out in the *Bhagavad Gita*, were Arjuna's major arc is to balance his duties and his actions. Although Arjuna projects his struggles through his conversation with Krishna, the struggle is deeply internal and bears a striking resemblance to the greater jihad within the personal battles of Muslims. The balance of justice also recalls the balance of the *Dao* (道) of ancient Chinese philosophy. Islam demonstrates a special elegance in not only its ability to derive similar conclusions as other schools of thought, but also to build on them in a way that leads towards a greater harmony and collaboration.

'Justice is a state of being, a condition of things being in their proper places. It is also the quality of human act', says the Malaysian philosopher, Syed Muhammad Naquib Al-Attas. Justice is active but it is more than that. It is both a completion and a project in development at the same time. A mutual understanding echoes in the teachings of Confucius. Despite being an intellectual adversary of Daoism, Confucius appeals to the metaphysical conundrum that arises in attempting to understand the Dao and uses this understanding as a mode to seeking truth, a metaphor for being a good person. *Junzi* (君子) can be translated as 'gentleman' or 'exemplary person', but is often mistranslated as 'sage'. To Confucius, to be a sage is a lifelong vocation – and a utopian ideal – that can never be attained in a human's lifetime (lest one lose the motivation to continue being good), but the *exemplary person* is one who tries to do what is right and works to correct past wrongs and is always constantly working to better himself or herself. Keeping with this, in regards to the knowledge required to uphold justice, Al-Attas appeals to the term *wuṣūl*, or arriving. The arrival intended here is not a final destination. Rather, it is an active, always ongoing process. The pursuit of justice never ends. An apt metaphor for *wuṣūl* is found in the Mike Oldfield composition *Tubular Bells*, originally recorded in 1972 using a 16-track tape recorder. But once a decade, Oldfield would re-record the tune as new instruments and new technology would allow him to meticulously continue perfecting the tune. As more techniques become available, presumably Oldfield will continue to tweak the song until it matches what he hears in his head.

So here we find ourselves in the midst of a pandemic with so much work to do. We have to realise that the project of justice will never be completed, we will always be arriving: from each subsequent analysis, from generation to generation, we will watch a rich tapestry weave itself in the work we do.

Each one of my stays in prison found me freed into an entirely different world. My first release took me from the turbulent 1970s into a hopeful, yet worrisome 1980s of growth, progress and neoliberal ecstasy. I went back to prison at the end of the 1990s where financial doom and the technological terror of the new millennium left the air nearly unbreathable. And my most recent release, only just over two years ago, finds me in a world ruled by the internet of things, social media, and the increasing digitalisation of our lives. And in just two years the world itself has been flipped on its head several times, struggling to keep up with simultaneous crises of nationalism, greed, xenophobia, and that's before we get to the economic rollercoasters and our present pandemic. I have grown rather accustomed to, nearly an expert on, change; and radical changes they have been indeed. Yet while the images may change, the underlying human suffering and injustices remain and needs to be continually stood against. Sources of evil are so powerful because they are advantaged in their ability to evolve and change. So, if we want justice in our futures then we too must adapt our notions. Or else we will lose sight of the faces of injustice standing right in front of us.

At this moment we have not just the immediate quandary that stands front and centre, the Covid-19 pandemic, but a simultaneous onslaught of compounding and complex crises that need to be approached and navigated simultaneously and with innovative and creative approaches. The exponential growth of inequalities and divides, the natural by-product of the global capitalist system, the rise of xenophobic sentiment within isolationist and nationalistic fervour, the disrupted lives of migrants seeking refuge from human violence and environmental disaster, the good, bad, and ugly of our digital futures, and, of course, climate change. This sample barely scratches the surface of all the crises we face both collectively and from country to country and life to life. We must heed the warnings of disastrous inequality exposed by the French economist Thomas Picketty in his book *Capital in the Twenty-First Century*. We need to be considering the reality of *The Age of Surveillance Capitalism* and our digital rights elucidated by Shoshanna Zuboff. We need to rethink our conventional notions of justice in a technologically driven 'age of extremes' as Mimi Sheller proposes in *Mobility Justice*. It is imperative that we seek green, sustainable ways forward to navigate climate change. Plus, there is a whole host of emerging crises on the horizon that we aren't currently thinking about as we are too busy dealing with what is already on our plates. What are we not thinking about? Are enough voices being heard? Are any being silenced? What is poverty today? We need to challenge our conventional definitions. Poverty now is also immobility. There is digital poverty too. As the great paradox of capitalism shows that while the rich get richer, it may be hard to conceptualise the poor getting poorer, but their right to the mechanisms of upward mobility get further and further from their grasp. And that is wrong. That is why we need justice for our times. For me it is personal. That is why the political party I helped found holds Justice as its namesake.

The justice we need now is not simply 'fairness' it needs to be about equity and we need to work out how to see it out in the real world. Justice is not about being impartial, but instead, being impartial to the truth, which does still persist in this world of fake news and alternative facts. And we must remain humble, for we may not have the right answer and even if we find an answer that works, we must not fly so close to the sun and assume it as some universal solution. We must not be led astray, thinking that justice arises through victories, this is the infection of neoliberal capitalism speaking through a corrupted notion. Justice is a balance and involves the efforts of the many. The just world we crave is aided in the formation of a global Convivencia. It is incumbent upon us, be we Muslim or not, for it is an objective for all humans to strive for, the alignment that puts all things in their right place. This starts with us not just living next to each other, but living by one another and dismissing false stereotypes and manufactured boogiemen.

In the guise of a pandemic, history has offered us a warning and a moment to pause and reflect. I pray this time we do not miss an opportunity to improve our condition and the condition of everyone else on this planet. If we do not think about our futures and attune our thinking, it will be too late and we will be left in a cell with no comfort but what comes from prayers. The dream is not a utopia. Suffice it to say it will not be easy. But democracy can be slow and can be messy, but such is compromise and peace.

Patience for now, but I have not stopped moving yet.

THE METAPHYSICS OF VIRUSES

Colin Tudge

The case for the prosecution seems open and shut. Viruses are life's disrupters – nature's spivs, gangsters, the ultimate parasites; dogging the lives of all other organisms through their single-minded yet mindless compulsion to replicate. They lack the metabolic wherewithal to carry out all of life's vital requirements and cannot reproduce unaided so they hi-jack the genetic apparatus of more complete creatures to do what's necessary, often causing havoc along the way: disease, suffering, death, pandemic, even extinction. In a theological vein, at least in some traditions, they might well be seen as the embodiment of evil.

But life is never quite so simple. Ghastly though their effects can be, at least from the sufferers' point of view, viruses, it now transpires, are essential players in what is often called 'the grand scheme of things'. Without viruses, as many biologists are now telling us, the rest of us – fungi, beetles, oak trees, human beings – would not exist. Perhaps there would be no life at all – or not at least, 'life as we know it'. In truth, the metaphysical concept that viruses most cogently illustrate is that of yin and yang: opposing qualities that between them make a whole.

The case for the prosecution

Scientists first showed in the 1890s that viruses exist and it has taken 130 years to get a handle on what they really are, how they operate, and their roles in the lives of other organisms and in the global ecosystem – aka 'Gaia'. They still raise huge problems for science – not just in molecular biology and medicine but, more broadly, in the still-infant science of ecology. Yet the issues they raise extend beyond biology and into metaphysics; with huge implications for moral philosophy and for political and economic theory. In short, whatever else they may be, viruses are salutary. They inform our *attitude* to life and to ourselves. The questions that apply to them – what is their status, their *role* in the global ecosystem? How do they fit in? – apply at least equally to human beings.

Physically, viruses are packages of nucleic acids, DNA or RNA, single-stranded or double-stranded, enclosed in a protein membrane, sometimes with some lipids (fat). Thus they contain some of the control mechanisms of life though without the apparatus that goes with it. This they borrow from their host – which may be any other life form: any animal (including us), plant, fungus, protist, or bacterium – for viruses are many times smaller than bacteria (which in turn, in general, are many times smaller than the cells of plants or animals).

Viruses as a whole do not constitute what taxonomists would call a 'true taxon' or a 'clade': a group of related organisms with a common ancestor, like tigers, or oak trees, or mammals or fungi. Rather they are a collection of clades, which seem to have arisen independently of each other, in different ways. Some – conceivably – are simply primitive: quasi-life forms that arose out of non-living materials in the way that *bona fide* organisms in general are assumed to have arisen. But if that is the case, they could not have arisen until *after* other life-forms had appeared, since they cannot survive (if survival is the word) *except* by hijacking the genes and metabolism of existing creatures. Some kinds may have derived from *transposons*, aka 'jumping genes': packages of DNA that naturally move around within the genomes of creatures like us and plants. Transposons that broke free of their parent genome, and acquired a bit of protein protection, would be *de facto* viruses. Some perhaps derived from *plasmids*: bits of DNA that reside within the cytoplasm of the cell, rather than the nucleus. There is some evidence for each of these possibilities in different groups.

However viruses arise, once they have broken free they must find new hosts, which they enter in all kinds of ways: via water or food; in air-born droplets; by direct physical contact; or introduced by some vector. Sap-sucking aphids are prime carriers of plant viruses. Some viruses can infect a whole range of other species while others are highly specialised. Often we find small families of closely related viruses, each with their preferred host. Thus the genus *Morbilivirus* includes the agent of measles in humans, which can also infect monkeys and apes; and also the agent of distemper in dogs and other carnivores; and the kind that causes phocine distemper of seals, which also occurs in dolphins; and the agent of rinderpest, otherwise known as cattle plague, in cattle and other hoofed animals. Some viruses, like those of flu and the common cold, rapidly evolve to produce new strains that may re-infect populations that had developed immunity to earlier strains; or mutate into new forms that may cross erstwhile species barriers. A whole catalogue of viruses also lay waste a great array of agricultural and horticultural crops, from barley and maize to cauliflowers, tobacco, and tomatoes. Others, known as phages (literally, 'eaters') are the scourge of bacteria, the ultimate illustration of Augustus de Morgan's observation that 'Great fleas have little fleas upon their backs to bite 'em, and little fleas have lesser fleas and so *ad infinitum.*' But it isn't quite *ad infinitum.* Viruses are the end of the line.

Sometimes the invading virus not only causes illness, often severe or lethal, but may also affect the behaviour of the host in ways that favour its own transmission. Thus rabies can affect all warm-blooded animals, both mammals and birds. Humans commonly catch it from dogs. Some infected dogs become hyper-aggressive – the 'mad dog' of myth and of fact that foams at the mouth and bites anything that moves indiscriminately. Everyone steers clear of mad dogs. Sometimes, however, infected dogs become over-trusting and over-friendly. They approach human beings for a cuddle and a pat, and lick their hands and faces; apparently sweet but potentially fatal. Rabies is no longer indigenous in Britain though it may be brought in from time to time with pets, and perhaps in bats, some of which can cross the English Channel. But wherever you are, beware over-friendly stray dogs.

Some viruses may lay entire populations to waste, sometimes to the point of extinction. For centuries, smallpox was the scourge of humankind. In India, in past times, men and women preferred to find wives or husbands who were pockmarked, because this indicated previous infection and hence immunity (the variola virus of smallpox induces very strong immunity). Smallpox was eradicated in the wild by the 1970s through a truly heroic, global vaccination programme, showing what human beings can achieve when they work together. Yet in the preceding seventy-odd years of the twentieth century, variola is estimated to have killed 200 million people. Measles was a prime cause of infant mortality among malnourished children in Africa and elsewhere before an effective vaccine became available. In

Britain when I was a boy (in the 1940s and 1950s) measles was regarded as a 'common childhood disease', more or less routine, yet even here it was a prime cause of non-congenital blindness and deafness. In my childhood days in Britain the great spectre, feared by all mothers, was polio, but effective vaccines were created in the 1950s and 1960s and the World Health Organization hopes to eradicate the disease entirely by 2023 – although, of course, Covid-19 has been a massive distraction which surely will delay things, and perhaps will enable polio to break out again. The 'Spanish' flu epidemic of 1918–19 infected about 500 million people worldwide (a third of the total population) and killed an estimated 50 million; more than twice as many as were killed in World War I (though World War II killed 80 million). By the end of November 2020, the Covid-19 pandemic has killed over a million people worldwide but if left unchecked it could surely, over time, kill more than 100 million. (Bubonic and related forms of plague, which is estimated to have killed 30–60 per cent of Europe's population in 1348–49, is caused by a bacterium).

Mercifully, many epidemics (pandemics are mega-epidemics) are self-limiting. Measles is so transmissible and potentially lethal (particularly among the malnourished) that it quickly infects *most* of the susceptible people in any one population. But the body does mount a very effective immune defence against it so those who recover are henceforth immune – so that soon, the unlucky ones in the population are dead and those left alive are immune. So the virus runs out of hosts and then it goes locally extinct – though it may still remain in other populations and so may re-infect when a new generation arises of children who are not immune. Measles cannot persist long term in small isolated populations.

Sometimes, though, a virus finds alternative host species that are less susceptible and it then may linger within them at a low level – and continue to infect other hosts that are more susceptible. Thus phocine distemper is highly transmissible and is very likely to kill common seals and if no other influences were at work it should quickly run through a common seal population and then die out, at least locally, like measles in humans. But the phocine distemper virus has less effect on grey seals and so may continue among them at low levels and continue to infect new generations of common seals. Covid-19 (a coronavirus) is potentially as dangerous as it is precisely because it is *not* as lethal as measles; it kills only a small proportion of those infected; it may not induce a very powerful immune response in its hosts; and we now know that it can and does mutate into new forms. For us, the hosts, this is surely the worst of all worlds.

All in all, the case against viruses does indeed seem pretty conclusive. They are the villains of the biosphere: self-seeking killjoys. And yet ...

The upside

As the American science writer Rachel Nuwer reports in an article posted on the web on 8 June 2020, a whole host of modern biologists now assure us that while *some* viruses do such enormous and obvious harm to people, livestock, crops, and wildlife alike, *by far the majority do not*. Indeed, says Professor Curtis Suttle of the University of British Columbia, the percentage of viruses that cause problems for humans is 'statistically close to zero'. On the contrary, their net effect is decidedly beneficial to the whole, not to say essential. Says Tony Goldberg of the University of Wisconsin-Madison: 'If all viruses suddenly disappeared, the world would be a wonderful place for about a day and a half, and then we'd all die.'

The changing attitude towards viruses, along with a few other modern insights, is contributing to what might properly be called a 'paradigm shift' in the whole science of ecology: not just an expansion of existing ideas but a complete change of perspective. Thus, when I was at university in the early 1960s electron microscopes were already in use but ecologists by and large studied only those organisms that can be seen with the naked eye or with simple light microscopes. Birds, mammals, insects, and wildflowers were the stamping ground. Bacteria and other micro-organisms were of course recognised as pathogens and also as agents of decay and nitrogen fixation but viruses were hardly if ever mentioned in an ecological context. It was more or less taken for granted too that all food chains began with plants or green 'algae' (many of which are not classified as plants). The overall structure of ecosystems was taken to be determined from the bottom up: particular kinds of soil allowed some plants to grow but not others; the kind of plants that grew determined what herbivores would be present; and the nature of the herbivores determined what predators would flourish. It all seemed very logical and obvious.

Now, however, it is clear that the influence spreads both ways; top down as well as bottom up. Thus, to take a classic modern example, the wolves in wild ecosystems largely determine not only the numbers of deer but also their behaviour – whether for example they dare to spend time grazing by rivers and lakes, where the fodder is lush but the predators lie in wait. This profoundly affects which plants grow where. Also obvious now is that the very smallest organisms – bacteria, archaeans, *and viruses* – are huge players in all the world's ecosystems. In their capacity as pathogens they largely determine which plants, animals, and fungi can flourish – and how numerous they can become. Rabbits are key herbivores but their numbers are regulated up to a point by the myxoma virus (myxomatosis). Rabies in recent years has threatened the dwindling populations of African wild dogs – key predators. And so on.

Most important of all though, probably, is the impact of phage viruses on bacteria – which in turn, taken all in all, probably influence the ecology of the whole world more than any other organisms. Indeed says Tony Goldberg (as reported by Rachel Nuwer), phages are 'the major predators of the bacterial world'. Every day, in the world's oceans, viruses kill an estimated 20 per cent of the micro-organisms – which between them account for more than 90 per cent of the total oceanic biomass; and this 20 per cent includes 50 per cent of the ocean's bacteria. Since the micro-organisms in the oceans produce about 50 per cent of the oxygen dissolved in the world's waters and in gaseous form in the atmosphere, this daily mass wipe-out may not seem particularly desirable. But, says Curtis Suttle, 'If we don't have death, then we have no life, because life is completely dependent on recycling of materials'. Viruses, in short, are key re-cyclers.

Viruses aren't just killers. However, increasing evidence is revealing more and more interactions with other creatures that help those creatures to survive. So it is that cattle and other ruminants rely on bacteria in their voluminous stomachs to digest the cellulose in grass and other vegetation – and it now seems that those bacteria in turn are abetted by viruses. The break-down products of cellulose are the chief course of energy for ruminants and other big herbivores (elephants, horses, rabbits and the rest) but without their (virus-assisted) gut bacteria the cellulose would remain 'inert' and provide no energy at all. Medical research is revealing more and more beneficial effects in humans too. As Rachel Nuwer reports, GB virus

C, a distant, non-pathogenic relative of the dengue fever virus, may delay the progression of HIV in AIDS victims; and it also apparently improves the life chances of people with Ebola. Herpes infection seems to make mice less susceptible to some bacterial pathogens, including the ones that cause bubonic plague (which is still a problem in some countries) and listeria (a cause of bacterial food poisoning which is the particular bane of cheese-makers). Such observations could conceivably lead to useful therapies or preventives. Phages in particular have obvious therapeutic potential, which is attracting more and more attention as greater numbers of bacteria become resistant to more and more antibiotics. In the 1920s, scientists in the Soviet Union did a lot of research on phage therapy, so Nuwer tells us. All in all, it seems, a great many relationships between viruses and hosts, including human hosts, are not so much destructive as symbiotic.

Even more intriguing though is the role of viruses in shaping the genetics and hence the evolution of the creatures they infect – which could include each and every species on earth. Viruses pick up genes from their hosts and may insert them into the genomes in new hosts – 'horizontal transmission' – both within and between species. It seems indeed that eight per cent of our own DNA was brought to us by viruses. Evolution, so Charles Darwin told us, *depends* on novelty; a constant supply of new characteristics. Darwin knew nothing of genes but the past hundred years of biological research have shown that this novelty is supplied by genetic mutation. Now, though, it seems that novelty is also brought in by viruses – as genes that may be transferred from other species or may conceivably have arisen within the virus vector itself.

'Genetic engineers' make use of similar mechanisms to transfer genes between species. Many (including me) believe that genetic engineering of crop plants and especially of livestock is deeply pernicious – not least because it has drawn attention and funding away from the traditional techniques which, often, with little economic help, would generally serve the world much better; and thereby serves also to transfer power and wealth from the many (the world's many millions or billions of small farmers) to the few (corporate executives and shareholders). On the plus side, however, genetically engineered micro-organisms are already yielding new generations of vaccines. The techniques of gene transfer and gene editing too, and the study of viruses themselves, have long been helping the science of molecular biology to advance by leaps and bounds. This is a huge contribution to theoretical biology in general – 'knowledge for its own sake', and the practical possibilities, generically labelled 'biotech', seem endless, in all fields, not least in conservation biology. Science does not have to be, and certainly should not be, the handmaiden of big business.

All this – the changing face of ecological science in general; the ecological significance of microbes in general and of viruses in particular; the multiple roles of viruses within individual organisms – not just as agents of disease; the undoubtedly profound influence of viruses in evolution; and, finally, the role of viruses in advancing molecular biology and biotech – has profound metaphysical implications. After all, as Karl Popper pointed out (not least in his 'intellectual autobiography', *Unended Quest*), matters that can be studied by scientific experiment can nevertheless be matters of metaphysics.

Viruses and metaphysics – and the way the world is run

The constant flow of genes between organisms – often very different organisms, not closely related at all – reinforces one of the key concepts of metaphysics: that of *oneness*. To be sure, the idea of 'oneness' has many connotations, mostly of a spiritual kind, but the sharing of genes should surely be seen as a physical manifestation of the idea. Modern taxonomists, essentially taking their lead from Darwin, tend to depict each lineage of creatures as a twig on one giant 'tree of life' that is rooted in some long-gone common ancestor who lived nearly four billion years ago. As time has passed, so the general notion has it, evolution has ensured that the descendants of this primordial creature became more and more different from their shared ancestor and from each other. But now it is known that within some lineages at least – particularly bacteria and plants – hybridisation between different species is common; and sometimes – fairly often in plants – the hybrids are fertile, and so they may evolve as new species that *combine* the qualities of their once disparate parents. The constant to-ing and fro-ing of viruses, potentially between each and every one of them, is another way of mixing the attributes of creatures that once had seemed entirely separate. Indeed, to borrow a thought from the seventeenth century cleric and poet John Donne, no creature is an island. Each of us is part of a far greater whole.

The key concepts of metaphysics are at the core of all religions – and importantly, although the fact is not generally acknowledged, they spill over into politics and economics. Thus the modern world is dominated in particular by the offshoot of capitalism known as 'neoliberalism': the idea that the world's economies should be built around the so-called 'free market', which really means unfettered commerce. The market is supposed to be maximally competitive – all against all and the competition is as ruthless as is necessary to generate the most wealth and come out on top. Moral justification for what may seem like organised viciousness (for those neoliberals who care to waste time on moralising) is derived in large part from a serious misreading of Darwin. In his seminal *Origin of Species* of 1859, Darwin argued that competition among organisms in the wild is what leads to natural selection and hence to evolutionary change. Competition in short is nature's way, and without it we would still be bacteria, if indeed we ever got that far. Twenty years before *Origin of Species,* Alfred (Lord) Tennyson wrote very resonantly of 'nature red in tooth and claw'. In the 1860s, Herbert Spencer summarised natural selection as 'survival of the fittest'. The preacher in *Ecclesiastes* tells us that 'the fight is not to the strong' – but the word has got round, helped by Tennyson and Darwin and miscellaneous intellectuals, that it very definitely is. This too is a common thread in moral philosophy, albeit a dubious one, that what is natural is therefore *right*. Thus the ultra-competitive, 'free' market, producing an elite of super-rich who play the commercial game well, is held in essence to be 'natural' – reflecting nature itself – and therefore the way of the world and therefore OK.

But Darwin was a truly great biologist and he also noted – he wrote about it at length – that nature is often cooperative and that individual animals often behave altruistically even though they receive no instruction either in religion or in moral philosophy. Now, with another 150 years of natural history behind us, we can see at least with unblinkered eyes that nature is *at least* as cooperative as it is competitive. Indeed a little thought tells us that unless nature was *more* cooperative than competitive there could be no cohesion. Ecosystems would fall apart. Indeed, individual organisms would fall apart because all organisms are cooperatives of different molecules, often with very different origins, working together. Thus I have been arguing of late – not least in the recently published *Why Genes are Not Selfish and People are Nice* – that what is now called 'Darwinism', or at least (in its various altered forms) is known as 'Neodarwinism', should be called 'Metadarwinism', where 'meta' means 'beyond'. The neoliberal economy in truth is metadarwinian. But the idea that nature is just one long, ruthless punch-up is not what Darwin said at all. It is not good biology – and even if it was, that would not mean that it was good morality.

Instead (as I suggest in my forthcoming book, *The Great Re-Think*) nature and indeed the universe as a whole are far closer in spirit to the Buddhist conception of *dharma*: the idea of universal harmony. The moral implication of this is that we, thinking human beings, should consciously try to contribute to that harmony. Whatever detracts from the harmony – as the prevailing political-economic madness of maximal competition certainly does – is destructive and bad. In short, the claim that neoliberalism is 'natural', that it imitates the ways of the world, is simply untrue, and the idea that it is therefore morally acceptable is bad biology and even worse moral philosophy. We need, in absolute contrast, to root the economy in cooperation. In the world's all-dominant business schools competitiveness is seen as the greatest of virtues. It is, in truth, a huge mistake; perhaps the single greatest cause of the world's present ills.

So what has all this got to do with viruses? Well, if viruses really were the ultimate spivs and destructors, they would strongly challenge the idea of the Dharma. They would reinforce the metadarwinian/neoliberal conceit that nature is a ruthless punch-up and that every other conception of it is just wishful thinking. But when we look at the biology of viruses in the round, we see that they offer no challenge at all. They are essential players in a global ecosystem that, despite the all-too obvious skirmishes, is fundamentally cooperative.

One last point, again of a metaphysical nature. The biological examples cited here, wondrous though they are, are only a small fraction of what is known (whatever 'known' may mean). But current knowledge in turn is a very small fraction indeed of what is going on in the world. We are only just beginning to glimpse the many roles that viruses play in human biology – and not simply as agents of disease – although humans are the best studied creatures of all. Goodness only knows what else is going on in nature, or has gone on in the past, and all of it may influence our lives one way or another. Indeed we have no idea, even to within orders of magnitude, how many different kinds of virus there are, and still less idea of how they operate. Come to that, we have very little idea how many species there are of *any* organism. About two million have been described but some estimates say 30 million and if we include bacteria it could be 100 million. As a conservative guess, biologists tend to suggest there are probably about eight million, of which *most* are completely unknown. Multiply the number of species there are by the number of possible interactions between them and we get to the kinds of numbers that make the breathtaking statistics of astronomy seem trivial. But perhaps that is progress of a kind. After all, according to Socrates, wisdom begins when we start to appreciate the extent of our own ignorance.

Ignorant though we are and must always be – for omniscience is not within our gift – we are part of nature's melee and must do our best to live within it. Very obviously, given the vastness of our ignorance and the poverty and uncertainty of our knowledge, we should proceed with caution. Instead we assume, or allow our 'leaders' to assume, that we can bend nature to our will, or indeed to the whims of fashion. This is hubris of the grossest kind – which the old Greeks recognised as the greatest folly and indeed the greatest sin of all. Right now, Covid-19 is running away with us – not least in the US and Britain which have the most advanced science and technology in the world but have also elected vainglorious governments that have been altogether too confident. Either they denied the significance of the virus, as Trump did; or they assumed they could control it – and all of nature – at will; and/or they decided that a mere pandemic should not get in the way of economic 'growth'. All this is ideological dogma and hubris writ large.

Covid-19 is showing that wild nature must be taken very seriously indeed. More broadly, viruses as a whole in all aspects show us that if we give a damn about the world or indeed about ourselves then we need a whole new mindset. Whatever else they may be, viruses are certainly salutary.

FROM GOD TO GOD

Syed Nomanul Haq

How many brave horsemen and how many beautiful,
chaste women were killed in the valley of 'Amwās.
They had encountered the Lord, but He was not unjust
to them.
When they died, they were among the non-aggrieved
people in Paradise.
We endure the plague as the Lord knows, and we were
consoled in the hour of death.

Twelfth-century historian, Ibn 'Asākir

Primary Arabic sources tell us that around 638, a severe plague broke out in 'Amwās, the ancient Emmaus in Syria, resulting in massive fatalities among the soldiers of the Arab army. The caliph – more solemnly, the Rightly Guided Caliph – 'Umar ibn al-Khaṭṭāb, concerned about the safety of his commander Abū 'Ubayda, summons him to make his way back to Medina forthwith. But, then, knowing the firebrand commitment of the commander and his uncompromising zeal, the caliph acts pragmatically: he gives an alternative formulation to his purpose, sending the message that the commander is required for an 'urgent matter'. And yet, Abū 'Ubayda manages to sense the underlying intent of the caliph and refuses.

While one is tempted to pause over the political implications of this act of what may be called open insubordination on the part of an army, and over its meaning in terms of the non-autocratic nature of the caliph's governance, let's continue with the story. In order to withdraw Abū 'Ubayda from the plague-stricken region, Caliph 'Umar decides to travel towards Syria himself. He reaches the garrison post at a place called Sargh, and meets the military commander personally. Here a caliphal consultative council is set up to decide the matter, an exercise that ends in a cold deadlock. But reports tell us that the leaders of the tribe of Quraysh had definitive advice for the caliph – supporting his concerns, their counsel is to make the commander and his army depart from the infected area. Abū 'Ubayda protests, saying that this amounts to fleeing from the decree of God. 'Yes, but this is fleeing from the decree of God to the decree of God,' responds the caliph. Thereupon, the army withdraws from 'Amwās.

With its dual pull, this authentic story embodies a paradigm case of the normative Muslim dilemma concerning the approach to pandemics. To flee or not to flee was the resounding question here. And here we see an irony – the irony that there exists an apparent inconsistency in the famous three public health principles that are derived directly from canonical Hadith, and it is this inconsistency wherein lies the religious and legal legitimacy of both pulls at the same time. As the normative doctrine was developed over the centuries, in the Islamic tradition, both sides of interpretation – in favour of flight from the afflicted land, and prohibiting such flight – remain equally strong, often in the ideas of the selfsame sage.

Three principles echo in Muslim societies during the recurrent cycles of the Justinian plague, which marked the beginning of the first of the Old World pandemic of plagues. The seventh century 'Amwās plague being one of these. The same three principles are to be found throughout the centuries of the Black Death pandemic, all the way to our own times? They are all to be found in the *Book of Medicine* of the Bukhari collection. Here is the first one that seems, with hindsight, to constitute the ground of ante-Bukhari Abū 'Ubayda:

> Said the Apostle of God, upon whom be peace: 'If you hear of an outbreak of plague (*ṭā'ūn*) in a land, do not enter it. But if plague breaks out in a place while you are in it, do not leave that place.

The second principle is derived from the Hadith narrated by the Prophet's wife Ā'isha. Asked about plague, he informed her that

> Plague was a punishment that God used to send upon whomsoever He willed. But He made it a blessing (*raḥma*) for the believers. None among God's servants who remains patient in a land where plague has broken out, and considers that nothing will befall him except for what God has ordained for him, but that God will grant him a reward similar to that of the martyr (*shahīd*).

And as for the root of the third principle, we have this report, again in Bukhari's *Book of Medicine*:

> The Prophet, upon whom be peace, said: 'No contagion; no evil omen in the month of Ṣafar; and no evil screaming bird …'

Thus: (1) no flight from and no entry into the afflicted land; (2) plague is both a blessing and a punishment – *raḥma* and martyrdom for the believers, chastising torment for others; and (3) no contagion. To wit, these are the three Hadith-derived guiding precepts for pandemic management as they are understood by the largest segment of the Muslim community. It would appear that, indeed, the whole religious and legal and social history of majority Muslim attitude to deadly disease outbreaks revolve around this tripartite core.

And, as noted, there seems to be an internal tension here, a tension that has been smoothed out in creative ways as we witness in the wise and strategic response of the caliph to the protesting commander. If one remains in the afflicted area, that is God's decree; and if one moves away, that too is God's decree. The implication seems to be that one acts pragmatically as reason (*'aql*) would suggest; not blindly, as swaying emotions would tempt.

We have an illustrative case of the Prophet's Companion (*Ṣaḥābī*), Abū Mūsā al-Ashar'ī (d. 672), the governor of Kufa. It is reported by the historian Ibn Kathīr (d. 1373) that a few friends called upon the governor while someone in his household was infected with plague. He instructed the visitors not to stay with him, advising them to move to a healthier region, to a less populated open area and gardens. According to the Companion, Ibn Kathīr writes, it is commonly believed that if one stays in a plague-stricken region, one would die; and again, the Companion reminds his visiting friends of the general belief that if one stays in the afflicted region and gets infected, he would have been saved if he had fled. Here Michael Dols, the historian of Islamic medicine, comments: 'Implicit in this story is not only the common practice of fleeing the disease but the recognition of contagion despite the fact that the Prophet had denied the pre-Islamic belief in contagion. The pragmatic intention of the prohibition against flight may have initially been to prevent the spread of contagious diseases.'

In contrast, one also recalls the account of the early-eighth-century Umayyad caliph 'Umar ibn 'Abd al-'Azīz when a devastating plague broke out in Syria and Iraq. The caliph was advised by his lieutenants to withdraw to a disease-free area, while being reminded of his predecessors who used to move to the open deserts in order to protect their health and to save themselves from plague. The Umayyad ruler is reported by the fifteenth/sixteenth century historian Suyūṭī to have responded passionately and categorically: 'By God, if you know I fear one day other than the Day of Judgement, then do not comfort my fears.'

Indeed, there did exist much controversy among Muslims concerning the correct understanding of the three normative plague directives. We have, in fact, a preserved text dating from the ninth century that surveys the range of these disagreements, a reliable text written by the famous scholar and literary critic Ibn Qutayba. With the self-evident title, *On the Differing Interpretations of Hadith,* the author discusses comprehensively the contentious issue of the Prophet's guidance regarding pandemics and contagion.

But controversies and differences of opinion can also yield happy results, providing a productive soil for innovative resolutions; indeed, the joy of studying human history is that it often shows us a string of paradoxes. What we actually see in the Islamic world in its days of pandemic havoc is a creative tension arising out of the contrariety of opinions. Why would an affliction, excruciating and intensely tragic in actual daily human experience, descend upon believers in the first place? Since there was no consensus of opinion in this matter, it blocked the possibility of a firm and single ideological basis for social activism. We should note this as a highly significant historical fact since it contrasts sharply with the case of the Christian world of Europe during the deadly Black Death years. In this latter case, it was practically a universal belief of the Church that the pandemic is God's overwhelming curse and punishment for our sins; this belief had risen to the status of an orthodoxy.

And so the Black Death was explained all around the continent in messianic, apocalyptic, and chiliastic terms, engendering characteristic social and religious movements and attitudes that do not have a parallel in Islam. Given the doctrinal disagreements, and given the absence of an institution equivalent to that of the Church that would promulgate any expiatory social acts, movements such as that of the Flagellants, which began in the mid-thirteenth century, could not have arisen among Muslim peoples. Here was a movement grounded upon the general and stable Christian belief that mortification of the flesh was the appropriate penance for our sins. Let's listen to the British historian Philip Ziegler:

> As the fervour mounted the messianic pretensions of the Flagellants became more pronounced. They began to claim that the movement must last for thirty-three years and end only with the redemption of Christendom and the arrival of the Millennium.

Notwithstanding some early fringe elements and some minority groups that arose in earnest and became important some two centuries after 'Umar ibn al-Khaṭṭāb, messianic movements and apocalyptic communal visions did not take root in the larger bulk of the Islamic milieu. Again, there was no ecclesiastical institution in the vast Muslim mainstream to direct and oversee any mass-scale display of redemptive rituals. Certainly, special kinds of prayers and supplications were recommended to dispel natural disasters, but these were performed individually, in households, or in local neighborhoods, not in street throngs nor in public squares.

Let's continue briefly in this comparative mode. Scholars have characterised the general European Christian reaction to the Black Death as one of profound fear, guilt, and pessimism. The pandemic was something macabre – gruesome and morbid, requiring extreme collective penance. All of this yielded what the celebrated English historian of witchcraft Hugh Trevor-Roper has called a European 'stereotype of fear' – we are told that the 'collective emotion played upon a mythology of messianism, anti-Semitism, and man's culpability for his sins'. Note anti-Semitism here. Now the question that reverberates in the chamber of history is, why was there no corresponding phenomenon in the Islamic milieu?

Most intriguingly, the answer lies in the internal tension of Muslim normative sources, and this is what I meant by calling it a creative tension. Plague was both a punishment and a blessing; a calamity as well as God's mercy (*raḥma*). Significantly the word *raḥma* in the particular Hadith is the same word that the Qur'an uses for the Prophet himself. This establishes a metaphysical equivalence between prophecy and natural affliction, affliction that God sends to his creatures. And more, elevated to the lofty rank of the martyr is the one who succumbs to it. Michael Dols recognises this feature of the Islamic religious and legal environment loudly, calling it 'unique':

> The claim for mercy and martyrdom was a major theological invention of Islam and is, to my knowledge, unique to Semitic religions. In the variable list of five Muslim martyrdoms, death by plague and by battle are always included; both are equal in God's favour and the believer is assured of reaching paradise …

Another peculiarity is noteworthy in this connection. Pronouncing plague as God's punishment, the particular Hadith under consideration here – Bukhari 5734, quoted above, (a) does not single out any specific community that is the subject of this divine wrath. Moreover, it (b) speaks about plague-as-punishment in the past continuous tense ('God used to' [do this]). And when it talks about the elevation of plague victims to the glorious height of the martyr, (c) it does not refer to 'Muslims' or 'believers'; rather, the reference here is to a generality, namely, 'God's servant (*'abd*).'

The implications are far-reaching. By virtue of (a), no particular religious minority can be held responsible for the pandemic. The implication of (b) is a very happy one, namely, that plague descended 'upon whomsoever God willed' as His punishment, but only in the past, in the bygone days; indeed it is his mercy (*raḥma*) now. And, finally, it is perhaps legitimate to draw the (drastic) implication from (c) that God's reward is for the entirety of humanity, for His *'abd*, for all those who remain patient in the face of a painful death caused by plague. It seems that it is these implications that generated a kind of communal behaviour that is not characterised by gloom or fear or pessimism or persecutions or a sense of guilt or blame – there is, for example, no equivalent in Islamic history of the anti-Semitism that was unleashed in Europe during the Black Death.

The verses from the twelfth century historian Ibn 'Asākir – celebrating the affliction as promising a coveted reward, a reward that is not bounded within time, a reward that is unending and transcendental -– do not constitute a rare exception. This contrasts sharply and meaningfully with the European Christian case. We have a record of much Arabic poetry serving as celebratory expressions of the highest recompense awaiting the suffering of a victim, and of the opportunity provided by God for supplication and intimate prayers. All of this might save the victim from falling into a morbid despair and from the weakening of a belief in a compassionate God.

It is interesting that this communal attitude continues until this day during the recurring waves of our present pandemic. For instance, a self-identified Muslim publishing house, called Tazkiyah Publications, recently compiled a *Muslims' Covid-19 Handbook*, put together 'in consultation with senior scholars'. These consultants are not named. But the thrust of the handbook remains in perfect tune with and is practically a reproduction of classical Islamic normative plague literature. It quotes the same Hadith genre that speaks of the pandemic as a reward, and the succumbing victim as the one who will gain the glory of the martyr. The very first canonical Hadith quoted in this publication promises the glowing reward for 'the one' who has patience, and not (only) for 'the Muslim/believer' who has patience. This is a humanistic gesture, that seems to be integrated into the traditional Islamic ethos, even if the contemporary compilers are not conscious of it.

Returning to the story of Abu 'Ubayda in Syria. No matter how unwillingly, but eventually he had to follow the orders of the caliph and withdrew his army from 'Amwās and came to the highlands. But at a place called Jābiya his life was claimed by plague! It is reported by the redoubtable Ṭabarī that 'Umar appointed Mu'ādh ibn Jabal to assume the command of the army. But soon after his selection, we find out, Mu'ādh too succumbed to the pandemic; and moreover his son, who was supposed to substitute for his father, also lost his life. These deaths had a crucial consequence for Islamic political and dynastic history. Under dire circumstances of plague casualties, the caliph ordered 'Amr ibn al-Āṣ, the acclaimed 'conqueror of Egypt', to lead people to safety. Then, given the vacuum created, he appointed Mu'āwiya ibn Abī Sufyān as commander in Syria. This last step seems to be decisive: it provided favourable conditions for the foundation of the Umayyad Empire.

As for the Umayyads, they suffered heavy losses. We read in traditional Arabic histories that the caliph Mu'āwiya II died in 683, just a few months following the beginning of his rule. Caliph Marwān's life too was defeated by plague. Others among the ruling elite also fell victim. In Kufa, Ziyād ibn Abi Sufyān died in 673. The relatively long-reigning Umayyad caliph Hishām was known to be so concerned about plague that he left Damascus for the desert where he lived among the Bedouins at Ruṣafa.

The history of plague in early Islam is largely reconstructed from the writings of Arabic historians and chroniclers who lived through the Black Death or belonged to the late fourteenth and early fifteenth centuries. Among them is Ibn Khaldun who lived through the peak of the Black Death. This is the graphic picture he has painted for us:

> In the middle of the eighth [fourteenth] century, civilisation in the East and West was visited by a destructive plague which devastated nations and caused populations to vanish. It swallowed up many of the good things of civilisation and wiped them out. It overtook the dynasties at the time of their senility, when they had reached the limit of their duration. It lessened their power and curtailed their influence. It weakened their authority. Their situation approached the point of annihilation and dissolution. Civilisation decreased with the decrease of mankind. Cities and buildings were laid waste, roads and way signs were obliterated, settlements and mansions became empty, dynasties and tribes grew weak. The entire inhabited world changed. The East, it seems, was similarly visited though in accordance with and in proportion to (the East's more affluent) civilisation. It was as if the voice of existence in the world had called out for oblivion and restriction, and the world had responded to its call.

The early Muslim societies were struck by at least five famous cyclical waves of the Justinian plague, so we are informed by an important historian al-Madā'inī (d. 840) whose lost work has served as a major source for later histories such as the *Ta'rīkh* of Ṭabarī. If this is the case, then the Black Death was the sixth. This latter has its own communal, religious and legal peculiarities, a prominent one of these we should register in closing. It now seems that voices declaring the pandemic as God's punishment have become louder.

Thus we have Ibn al-Wardī. Witnessing mounting plague deaths around him in Aleppo during 1349, the chronicler prays beseechingly, 'we ask God's forgiveness for our souls' bad inclinations; the plague is surely part of His punishment'. But we note here a telling inconsistency, for in the next breath our writer calls the affliction God's mercy and martyrdom. Similar is the case of the Andalusi polymath Ibn al-Khaṭīb (1313–1374). Recognising empirical evidence, he argues strongly in favour of contagion; but again he does this with an eminent inconsistency, identifying at the same time divine mercy and martyrdom embodied in it. Indeed, one is tempted to make the observation here that Islamic intellectual history is often characterised by momentous paradoxes.

QADAR

Usama Hasan

Since the start of the global coronavirus pandemic, a particular hadith of the Prophet, found in the most authentic canonical Sunni collections, has been widely quoted. The Prophet is reported to have said: 'If you hear of plague in a land, do not travel there. If it occurs in your land, do not leave, fleeing from it.' This is extraordinary advice from the seventh century! An even more subtle insight is gained from a related story about Caliph Omar, who was travelling in an expedition to Syria from Medina. On the way, news reached the Caliph of the plague of Emmaus in Syria. He consulted his advisors. One of them testified that he had heard the above tradition of the Prophet. So, Omar announced that they would immediately return to Medina. Abu 'Ubaydah bin al-Jarrah, one of the Caliph's senior advisors, questioned Omar. Apparently he had not heard the hadith directly from the Prophet himself and was not convinced of its authenticity. 'Are we fleeing from the decree (*qadar*) of God?', he asked. Abu 'Ubaydah's fatalism was so strong that he favoured completing the journey and submitting to the will of God, even if that meant disease or death. But Caliph Omar replied: 'We are fleeing from the decree of God to the decree of God.'

In other words, Caliph Omar understood deeply that everything is the decree of God – this is a rather obvious consequence of a monotheistic belief in One, Omniscient God who knows the past, present and future.

The concept of *Qadr* or *Qadar* is a prominent theme in the Qur'an. Variously translated as Decree, Fate, Predestination, or Predetermination, it is also one of the most contested within Islam, right from its inception. Many hadiths record questions put to the Prophet about such matters. After his death, there appeared a group called the *Qadaris* (Free-Willers) who denied predestination completely and believed that humans had complete free will, otherwise human responsibility was impossible and heaven and hell made no sense. Many leading Companions, such as 'Abdullah the son of Caliph Omar, strongly condemned them as heretics. Later, a group known as the *Jabaris* (Determinists) appeared. They were the opposite extreme to the *Qadaris* and believed in total predestination: humans had the illusion of free will, but were effectively 'forced' (*jabr* or *jabar*) by Divine Omniscience.

Imam Ali's intervention in the controversy is rather instructive. '*Qadar*', he said cryptically, 'is God's secret in His Creation'. Muslims who criticise Christians for saying that the Trinity is a mystery, would do well to remember that Islam also has a mystery amongst its core beliefs, as illustrated by this quote. This core belief is most famously recorded in the first full hadith of *Sahih Muslim*, a long hadith that is actually there only in the context of condemning the Qadaris, since it includes the Prophetic teaching that one of the basic tenets of faith is 'to believe in *Qadar*, its good and bad'.

The leading Egyptian Sunni theologian Abu Jafar Ahmad al-Tahawi (843–933 CE) repeated Caliph Ali's aphorism verbatim in his concise *Creed ('Aqidah)* text, the most widely-accepted formulation of its type in Sunni Islam. Imam Tahawi also repeated the standard Sunni formulation of being balanced between the positions of *Qadar* and *Jabar*. The Sunni Ash'ari school of theology would later make a stunningly-honest admission: in their understanding, Sunnis are *Jabaris* (Determinists), intellectually speaking. However, it should be noted that Ash'ari determinism is not quite like modern scientific determinism. Ash'arism, in its doctrine of occasionalism, denies causality, believing that God is the cause of all things, and to attribute effects to secondary causes such as scientific laws is polytheism. But Ash'ari thought led to the practical Sunni and Sufi teaching of Ali Hujwiri (1009-1072), the celebrated South Asian mystic and teacher popularly known as Data Ganj Bakhsh, whose tomb is the famous Data Darbar in Lahore. In his *Kashf al-Mahjub (Unveiling of the Veiled)*, Hajwiri declares: 'Believe that everything is predetermined, but behave as though nothing is.' Ironically, the noted late physicist, Stephen Hawking, came to an identical conclusion based on scientific considerations.

One of the reasons that *Qadar* is so contested, quite apart from the basic underlying paradox of human free will within the realm of an Omniscient God, is that the word has so many senses and meanings in the Qur'an:

power, capability, and determination (in the strict sense of determining something). It is also associated with the greatest and most mysterious night of the year in the Islamic calendar: the Night of Qadar, usually associated with God, The Spirit and the angels during Ramadan – a time for intense worship. Perhaps the most relevant meaning of Qadar is measure or potential, as in a magnificent verse of Surah al-Ra'd (*Thunder*, 13:17) that begins: 'God pours down rain from the sky, so dry-valleys flow with water, each according to its potential (qadar) ...' The outer meaning of this verse is obvious. The inner meaning is that rain represents God's mercy and guidance that descends into the human realm, but each soul's uptake of these is limited to its potential. Spiritual journeys help to increase such potential of course, for life is a journey where one's potential may increase or decrease at any time.

As a lifelong student of Islamic scriptures and modern science, it is obvious to me that one of the meanings of *Qadar* is related to the nature of things (their potentials) and hence to the precise scientific laws that govern the physical universe. As the great mystic Ibn 'Arabi (1165-1240) observed, the 'Laws of Nature' that include the laws of science represent the operation or manifestation of the Divine Names. These include those related to *Qadar*, such as *Al-Qadir*, *Al-Qadeer* and *Al-Muqaddir*: the Powerful, the Omnipotent and the Determiner.

Caliph Omar's quip, 'we are fleeing from the decree of God to the decree of God', may be understood in a scientific sense as follows: entering a plague-ridden place subjects a person to the likelihood of being infected by a contagious disease – this is the decree of God because God has determined how diseases spread; but returning to a plague-free place is also the decree of God because God has determined that people will not be afflicted by a disease if its carriers, such as viruses or bacteria, are not physically present.

A related teaching is that from the Prophet himself. He was asked: 'O Messenger of God! Do you see the spiritual cures we use, the medicines by which we treat each other, the defences that we set up (against enemy attack) – do they repulse any of God's Predetermination (Qadar)?'. The Prophet replied: 'They are part of God's Predetermination (Qadar)'. In other words, parts of God's decree or determination (Qadar) work against other parts. In this hadith, medicine, both physical and spiritual, fights against disease, both physical and spiritual. Warfare proceeds according to Qadar also because God has decreed (via His Divine Names operating as laws of nature or science) that some people, technologies and strategies are stronger than others in various contexts.

A basic analysis of Islamic scriptures supports the common-sense view: Muslims should take maximum precaution against the Covid-19 coronavirus, and not be confused by incorrect, fatalistic or anti-science arguments, anti-vaccine propaganda, fake news of conspiracy theories, even if they are presented with a religious veneer. We must 'follow the science', whilst of course recognising that even scientists differ about complex, non-linear phenomena, with a firm belief that the laws of science that dictate disease and cure are themselves sacred and close to the Divine Presence.

'For every disease, God has sent down a cure' – another saying of the Prophet. It is up to us to find the cure via scientific research. Furthermore, the many categories of a *shaheed* or martyr, where both these words of Arabic and Greek origin respectively mean a 'witness' (to God or Truth), include those who sadly die in plagues. By now, we may well know of someone who has died from Covid-19. So we must stay safe, follow the precautions, pray that God enables the science of medicine to find a cure to defeat the science of the virus and, in worst-case scenarios, mourn our martyrs who return to God, their Source and Origin, to Whom we belong and to Whom we are returning.

VIRAL CORONA CAPITALISM

Vinay Lal

Let us be clear from the outset: if an argument is to be made for the exceptionality of the coronavirus pandemic in the experience of humankind, it must revolve around the fact that, for a period of between two and three months, there was a global suspension of economic activity on a scale previously unknown and indeed inconceivable even to the most radical or imaginative thinkers on the planet. There have been epidemics and pandemics in the past which doubtless affected trade, and in the last four decades the global or near global transmission of new infectious diseases have necessitated small-term closures of local economies, or some temporary restrictions on certain airline routes. But the flights that were suspended in May 2003 when the SARS outbreak occurred represented a miniscule fraction of global air traffic at the time, and even in February 2020 when only a few countries had suspended flights to and from China, Covid-19 had wrought by far greater economic loss than what the world suffered in 2003. By early May of this year, when global air traffic had been suspended for six weeks or more in most countries, the economic loss was of a magnitude that can only be described as incomprehensible. The singular fact is that no one really thought that it might be possible to shut down global aviation for such a length of time, close manufacturing plants all over the world, shutter shopping malls, empty out streets, cafes and restaurants, and keep billions of people off the streets and in 'lockdown' at their homes.

If, in our capitalist economy, homo sapiens is fundamentally homo economicus, what might be the implications of living in a time, and for a protracted period of time, when as human beings we ceased to be primarily economic agents? Some might quarrel with such a description and argue that supermarkets and food stores remained open, and that, in consequence of the shutting down of shopping malls and retail stores, the consumer economy merely shifted online. But any such argument can only be described as at best churlish. From the standpoint of those whose business it is to understand what the implications of the pandemic may be for small shopkeepers, chain clothing stores, department stores, mall owners, and, as in poorer countries, those who make their living as peddlers, owners of open air street stalls, vendors in public markets, and as craftsmen and technicians in dozens of trades, there are some vital questions about whether the livelihoods associated with such enterprises can be sustained in the present pandemic or in future pandemics of this kind. Questions of this kind, however, cannot be addressed only within the ambit of political economy. The future of the shopping mall, as an illustration, may also revolve around whether architecture can be adapted to a form of existence contingent upon the recognition that a coronavirus, or some other pathogen, is hovering round the corner.

The US, with 4.25% of the world's population, consumes about one fourth of the world's energy resources. Consumer spending accounts for 70% of the GDP (gross domestic product), but American consumers play a significant role as global consumers taking up, in 2018, a share of 15.2% of the global GDP adjusted for purchasing power parity (PPP). Their share of the global GDP has not declined much, being 15.8% in 2014, even as the consuming class in China and to a lesser extent in the other BRICS countries (Brazil, Russia, India, and South Africa) and other 'developing' nations has registered considerable growth. Even in circumstances which are not defined by a cataclysmic event of the magnitude of the pandemic, if the US heads into a deep 'recession', the rest of the world is very likely to follow in that direction. To that extent, apart from such considerations as the continuing allure of the greenback, the US remains the lynchpin of the global economic system. It is another matter that to a substantial portion of the world population, even the language of 'recession' is alien: it means something to those who have salaried jobs, and even more to that much smaller portion of the population who are invested in the stock market, but the greater majority of the world population lives on very little, often on hand-to-mouth budgets. In any case, for all these reasons and many more, among them the military prowess of the US, the unrivalled place of American universities taken as a whole in global higher education and more importantly, in the worldview of the middle class imaginary, and the cultural capital signified by Hollywood, American popular music, and a host of other phenomena, one can justify first turning to the US in an effort to comprehend some of the issues around political economy that emerge from the pandemic, even as I will advert to Europe, where most nations have registered significantly lower spikes in the ranks of the unemployed than in the US. More than anything else, the US is built on the house of capitalism, peopled by those who worship it, adore it, dream it, flaunt it, sell it, live by it, and kill in its name: America is the world's most preeminent shrine to capital.

Viral capitalism could only meet its match in a viral pandemic. Just what kind of discourse was being generated by the pandemic in the early days among economists, bankers, financial analysts, and corporate executives can easily be surmised from what I have hinted thus far. It all revolved around the performance of the stock market and the endless chatter, not much more interesting than that of baboons (except, and for good reasons, to primatologists) about whether the economy had slid into recession. On 16 March, just days after the WHO declared the coronavirus a pandemic, and as the virus toll soared, the Dow Jones Industrial Average fell by 12.93 per cent for its worst ever loss on a single day since the Great Depression of 1929, and it continued its steep decline over the next several days, and apparently trillions of dollars were wiped out with the market sell-off. And then much of this 'money' reappeared over the next several weeks, and billions and trillions were again lost, again regained. Meanwhile, to paraphrase T. S. Eliot, in the room the economists kept on coming and going, talking of the 'stock market' and 'recession'. That none of it matters to the 95 per cent or more of the people the world over who have nothing invested in the stock market is of no interest to economists since the profession prides itself on its mathematical model-building and insularity. But as the coronavirus pandemic has made it all too clear, the US stock market is akin to Pavlov's Dog: as hopes for a vaccine rise, sometimes based on nothing more than a claim advanced by Moderna, which was the front-runner among American pharmaceuticals in the chase for a vaccine, so does the market. Through the month of April, as New York slowly flattened the curve and deaths seemed to be declining in the US, the market became 'bullish'; then, in late June and July, as the virus swarmed over Arizona, Texas, Florida, and elsewhere, it started to limp. And on it goes – and all of this is apparently very interesting to the economists. If 20 million people in India were on the brink of starvation, or 20 per cent of Australia had burnt down due to raging wildfires, Dow Jones and the Standard and Poor Index would have nothing to say on either matter; neither would the economists. The economists long ago established their redundancy for, as the proverb goes, one can take the horse to a stream but one cannot make it drink.

But we may also enter into the heart of the enveloping darkness just through a brief consideration of two of the four headlines in the 'Business' pages of the *New York Times* of 15 July 2020. (There was a civilised time when newspapers did not have any business pages, let alone an entire section devoted to what William James in a letter to H. G. Wells of 11 September 1906 called the gospel or 'exclusive worship' of 'the Bitch Goddess Success', though recent generations are unaware of how such forms of barbarism slowly creep upon civilisation.) One headline states, 'Hero Raises by Retailers are Fading', and the article goes on to describe how, even as a record number of people in the US are being infected daily, nearly doubling to over 67,000 on 16 July from the 35,000 new confirmed cases on 23 June, American retailing giants have been withdrawing the 'bonuses' that they started handing out to workers at grocery or drug stores at the onset of the pandemic. These giant retailers, among them Walmart, Amazon, Target, and Walgreens, who are advised by an army of public relations officials, management experts, and 'diversity' consultants, understood that it was certainly expedient for them to join the national chorus in pronouncing grocery store workers as 'essential front-line' troops and 'heroes' when the initial chaos engendered by the pandemic set in.

One of the central planks in the strategy of maximising profits for shareholders and those in executive positions is to keep wages abysmally low, and then, when the occasion requires it, appear as paragons of generosity by handing out 'bonuses'. Thus, in the time of the pandemic, this bonus has generally entailed a raise of $1 or, as at Amazon, $2 an hour for minimum wage employees, though roughly in the same time period of three months the wealth of Amazon's founder and CEO, Jeff Bezos, increased by $48 billion to something like $175 billion. The *New York Times* report in question obscures the fact that all these corporations are egregious offenders in the matter of their treatment of workers employed at retail outlets and warehouses. When even a wholly mainstream magazine such as *Time* carries an article, titled 'They Treat Workers Like Robots', which describes the appalling working conditions at one of Amazon's 'Fulfilment Centres', it is a sure sign that there is no underlying commitment to the workforce. The pandemic has produced a new rhetoric of 'essential' workers and 'heroes', but all this is deployed merely to advance that shibboleth called 'corporate social responsibility' – and, needless to say, to generate more profits. Indeed, another article on the front page of the business section of the newspaper for the same day, which is not on the pandemic, is precisely on corporations seeking to become more respectable, and how else but by coming to this understanding: 'Why Not Treat Diversity Like a Profit?'

The next bolder headline from the business pages of the 15 July issue of the *New York Times* hogs far more attention: 'Lockdowns Eased, Europe Finds Plenty of Reasons to Shop Again'. The retail giants and corporate titans must perforce display the customary gestures of support for 'essential workers', as this is a cheap way of earning moral capital, but they have no interest whatsoever in their lives or welfare; the consumer, on the other hand, is all-important, or, as the business textbooks and marketing people emphasise, 'the consumer is king'. Many of the essential workers are, in fact, the very antithesis to the consumer. They have little disposable income, and sometimes live from one check to the next. The problem with the poor is that they are not good consumers; and to be poor is enough reason to be despised in America. So, no wonder, as the headline suggests, manufacturers and retailers have been watching anxiously the behaviour of consumers to see if they are ready to dig deep into their wallets, and it appears that businesses are pleased at what they are seeing: 'Consumers in Europe are going on a shopping spree as their economies reopen, offering hope that a fragile recovery from a deep pandemic-induced recession may be taking hold.' The argument that 'consumer spending is crucial to Europe's revival, accounting for more than half of its economic activity', is more than a trifle odd, since, by this reasoning, it is certainly critical in all developed and perhaps many developing economies. Why is consumer spending any more important in the revival of the economy in Europe than elsewhere in the world? In the

US, as I mentioned earlier, consumer spending constitutes 70 per cent of the GDP. It may not be the brief of the writer to consider why the idea of consumption weighs so heavily among those who are pondering what the coronavirus signifies to those with an interest in political economy, but the framework of the mainstream discourse effortlessly tags consumer inactivity to 'recession' and consumer spending to 'recovery'. The idea of consumption, if we adopt this line of reasoning, must remain fundamentally unquestioned. Two days later, not surprisingly, the business pages of the *New York Times* headlined another article, this one looking to the US rather than to Europe: 'Consumers Came Back. Is Recovery Sustainable?'That people may be thinking about more than just the stock market, recession, and consumption in the wake of the pandemic and the shuttering of the economy should be obvious. Among the working-class, whether employed in low-paying if steady jobs or, as is quite common in South Asia, Africa, Mexico, and South America, as daily wage-labourers, or slogging it out in the so-called gig economy, there are more pressing economic concerns and the fear is palpable. Initially, in many countries, it was uncertain who would pay for fourteen days of quarantine. Social distancing and the practice of quarantine is undoubtedly an unadulterated good from the standpoint of public health officials interested primarily in seeking to halt the transmission of the virus, but how does it help to put food on the table? The state may have assumed much of the responsibility of quarantine, but how far people will have gone into debt when they needed medical care will become clear over time. It is palpably clear that the poor, as described elsewhere in this book, are disproportionately affected by the disease, and many have been turned away from hospitals. The cloud of economic insecurity has always hung over the poor, and it has, with the spread of Covid-19, only got darker and larger. Most countries have adopted some relief measures, but countries with some notion of the collective good or, as in the case of the UK, with some demonstrable commitment to social welfare even as the self-employed and ethnic minorities remain vulnerable, have been more thoughtful about how they have attempted to minimise the corrosive social and economic aspects of the crisis. Even Britain's Conservative government showed perhaps more sensitivity than one might have expected in requiring employers to keep nonessential workers at home at up to 80% of their wages and capping payments to them at £2,500 a month. 'We are starting a great national effort to protect jobs', noted Rishi Sunak, the Chancellor of the Exchequer, in introducing the Coronavirus Job Retention Scheme, adding: 'We want to look back on this time and remember how in the face of a generation-defining moment we undertook a collective national effort and we stood together.' Most EU countries, as well as Canada, Australia, and New Zealand, have offered similar wage subsidies keeping non-essential employees at home for 65 per cent or more – as much as 90 per cent in Denmark – of their salary.

In consequence of these policies, EU countries were able to hold the jobless rate down to 6.5 per cent in May, and to 7.4 per cent in July. In India, by contrast, it went up from 8.7 per cent in mid-March to 23.5 per cent in May, though some studies claim that it is as high as 27 per cent. Prime Minister Modi announced on 12 May a relief package, dubbed as part of the Atmanirbhar Bharat Abhiyan [Making India Self-Reliant Mission] of ₹20 lakh crore, which can be rounded out to about $300 billion, constituting about 10 per cent of the country's GDP. This may sound reasonably generous for one of the poorest countries in the world, comparable as a percentage of the country's GDP to the initial $2 trillion 'stimulus' approved by the US Congress, but *the actual fiscal cost of the supposed 'relief package' is only one per cent of India's GDP*. Some of the relief measures had been taken before the announced package, many of the proposals are credit-focused, and as much as ₹8.04 lakh crore, or about 40 per cent of the proposed package, is merely additional liquidity that had been injected into the system by the Reserve Bank of India in the preceding three months. The government may claim that fiscal prudence is requisite in order for India to maintain sovereign credit ratings at a level that would still bring in foreign investment inflows, but the pressing requirement of the moment is cash transfers to the poorest and ensuring that food reaches all those who are hungry. But the government acts on the presumption that continued capitulation to neoliberal policies and striving to make India attractive to foreign investors outweigh the moral social pact that the state must make with its own people.

As is quite obvious, the implications of the suspension of months of economic activity are staggering and in some countries the situation, dire as it is, will continue to deteriorate. The WHO has warned repeatedly of the risks of mass food insecurity and famine in as many as thirty countries worldwide and reportedly by mid-April there were already a million people at the brink of starvation in as many as ten countries. The fifth edition of the monitoring report from the International Labour Organisation (ILO), dated 30 June 2020, begins with the grim observation that 'the vast majority, namely 93 per cent, of the world's workers continue to reside in countries with some sort of workplace closure measure in place'. The report is strikingly sensitive to the fact that the pandemic may set back efforts that have been years in the making in achieving gender parity, though the report does not elaborate upon the several dimensions to this very question. Women occupy a greater portion of lower-paid jobs than men, and have less job security than men; more of them live in poverty, especially as single parents with children, than do men, and this alone makes them more vulnerable. They constitute an overwhelming majority of healthcare workers, aside from physicians, and though the virus is far more lethal to men than it is to women, it is telling that a much higher number of female than male healthcare workers have been infected during the pandemic. In early April, 72 per cent of the infected healthcare workers in Spain were women; in Italy, that number was 66 per cent. They predominate industries and services, which shut down entirely during the pandemic, such as hospitality, hotels, and tourism, and not surprisingly over 55 per cent of the jobs lost in the US in April were held by women. In nearly every country of the world, women do more housework than men, even when they hold a salaried job, and childcare remains their responsibility. With schools shuttered and children at home, women's responsibilities have grown; some have had to relinquish their jobs, both to take care of children at home and elderly parents. In the words of one assessment of the gendering of the economic fallout of the pandemic in the US, it could 'scar a generation of working mothers'.

There can be little doubt that women in India will be even more adversely affected than women in the US, western Europe, or East Asia. Their situation is more precarious for a variety of reasons. India has one of the lowest participation rates of women in the labour market, and moreover this rate has declined over the last fifteen years even as it has grown in many other countries. Less than 21 per cent of Indian women participated in the labour market in 2019. As women become more educated, they are more likely to join the labour force; at the same time, in many communities, as incomes have risen and men have joined the ranks of the 'middle class', the women in these families have withdrawn from the labour force. In these households, the fact that a woman doesn't have to work is seen as a sign of upward mobility or affluence, though a more complete analysis of this cultural trait – visible among very well-to-do women married to extremely affluent men in the US – is beyond the scope of the present work and not entirely germane either. Economic precarity also suggests that more women will be forced into marriages that are not of their choosing – this is already an indubitable fact of Indian social structures, and Indian online matrimonial sites reported a surge of 30% in late April over the previous month. One can speculate that this is not merely because people looking for marriage partners cannot meet in person during the lockdown, but also because more parents will be pushing their young unmarried daughters into marriage – both to relieve their own economic distress and to secure, as they think, a home for their daughter in an uncertain future. If there is no emancipation or equality for women without economic freedom, where at least a woman herself desires such autonomy, then clearly the prospects for such a possibility stand eroded in the wake of the pandemic and the calamitous wounds inflicted on the economy. Two journalists may thus not be exaggerating in having written recently that the 'coronavirus economy' may be a 'devastating setback' for Indian women.

One could continue to marshal a wide array of figures, but ILO's own reports suggest, and as I have already pointed out, that the economic dimensions of Covid-19 cannot be captured only through statistics. The pandemic brings to the fore concerns that have agitated social justice activists and thinkers animated by questions of equity for years. For example, just as each state is called upon to do something for the poor and for ethnic minorities who are at greater risk, are not the rich states called upon to assist, more so than in 'ordinary' times, countries whose health systems are likely to be completely overwhelmed if the spread of the virus is not contained? There is the additional issue, with which I will conclude, revolving around the question of capitalism, and this in turn necessitates a slightly closer look at the circumstances that have facilitated the transmission of the virus worldwide – the globalist's dream! We may begin with this fact: around 20 July, as this is being written, the three countries with the largest number of infected people are the US, Brazil, and India. Might there be something in common between these countries? The answer is far from being self-evident even though some commentators have suggested that countries with authoritarian leaders, a characterisation that seems apt of these three countries, have fared poorly. Yet it is Xi Jinping's very authoritarianism that is thought to have made it possible to contain the pandemic in China; similarly, Turkey's Recip Erdogan is no novice in ruling with a firm hand, and the country seems to be on the path of flattening the curve.

A more plausible interpretation would have us consider the nature of healthcare in the US, Brazil, and India. The two largest democracies in the world quite possibly have the most chaotic healthcare delivery systems in the world; in one word, what characterises healthcare is the *privatisation* of what in most civilised societies is largely the responsibility of the state. The US has been singular among industrialised nations in not having universal health coverage, though the Affordable Health Care Act, known by the shorthand 'Obamacare', sought to extend coverage by opening up insurance marketplaces and making health insurance mandatory. This brought the percentage of those who were uninsured down to 8.5 per cent in 2018 from 13.3 per cent in 2013, the first year when Obamacare took full effect. Healthcare expenditures per capita are significantly higher in the US than in any other country and medical costs, including drugs, are similarly out of reach for all but those on generous employer-paid or private plans for which the premiums are exceedingly high. Only 21 per cent of hospitals are state-run. In India, the story is a similar one of lack of a uniform healthcare system and systematic neglect of public health, but in all other respects the situation is far more grim than in the US. The story of the precipitous decline of healthcare for all but a small portion of the population that may be described as belonging to the middle strata of the 'middle class' or above is perhaps best captured in this startling figure: only 1.15% of India's GDP is devoted to public spending on healthcare, as opposed to the worldwide average of 8.5%, 8% in the US, 11% in Germany, and 23% in Switzerland. India spends 4.2% of its GDP on private healthcare, twice the percentage spent in Germany, UK, France, and most of the EU countries, but just under half of the 8.8% of the GDP that goes towards private health spending in the US. An overwhelming eighty-two per cent of Indians have to draw exclusively on their own funds for healthcare. In India and the US, the poor are simply left to fend for themselves.

Brazil would not appear to fit into this picture. The 1988 Constitution of Brazil defines healthcare as a universal right and a responsibility of the state, and the authors of a very recent and exhaustive 2019 *Lancet* study, while recognising some of the shortcomings of the healthcare system in the country, are categorical in stating that 'Brazil has achieved nearly universal access to healthcare services for the population'. There have been impressive gains: life expectancy increased from 65.34 years at birth in 1990 to 75.20 years in 2015, and in the same period access to sanitation went up from 66.6 per cent to 82.8 per cent. But it is this last figure that should make us pause, as it shows clearly that 17.2 per cent of Brazil's 205 million people are still without access to proper sanitation which is fundamental to public health. The authors themselves point to 'geographical inequalities', but we can be more blunt in admitting that the poor and racial minorities in Brazil, as in other countries, suffer disproportionately to their numbers in the matter of healthcare. The state may in principle commit itself to constitutional rights for all of its citizens and at the same time may carry out policies that are by design detrimental to the well-being of a certain class of its citizens.

To this end, another comparison becomes even more instructive, one which enables us to view the pandemic coursing through Pakistan, India's neighbour to the west, and Bangladesh, its neighbour to the east. The three countries have a shared history: Pakistan was carved out of India in 1947, and advocates of independence in its eastern half were able to prevail in 1971 giving birth to Bangladesh. The following table, drawn from data available on the Johns Hopkins University Coronavirus Dashboard, shows where matters stood on 19 July:

	Population	Cases	Deaths
India	1.366 Billion	1,077,781	26,816
Pakistan	216.56 Million	263,495	5,568
Bangladesh	163.05 Million	202,066	2,581

Pakistan's Prime Minister Imran Khan crowed on Twitter about his country's success on 17 July arguing that 'Pak[istan] is amongst the fortunate countries where Covid-19 cases in hospitals, esp[ecially] in intensive care & death rate have gone down, unlike in our unfortunate neighbour India'. The figures somewhat belie his claims. With almost a fourth of the total number of cases in India, and almost a fifth of the number of deaths, Pakistan's case rate per million is 56 per cent higher than India's; moreover, Pakistan has conducted fewer than 10 per cent of the number of tests conducted by India, and the WHO has advised Pakistan that it must ramp up testing and that it did not meet any of the conditions the WHO set out in mid-April for ending a lockdown. What is most pertinent, for the purposes of my argument, is that the state of the healthcare infrastructure in Pakistan is roughly comparable to what it is in India, and similarly Pakistan has an abysmal record in healthcare delivery for the poor. It is Bangladesh's record, however, which is illuminating in suggesting that its investment in public health infrastructure and 'development' in the ordinary sense – as manifested by increased spending for the health of women and children, enhanced literacy rates especially for women, attentiveness to nutrition, hygiene, and sanitation, among others – is why some countries have been more successful in mitigating and then containing the effect of the coronavirus than other countries. There is now insurmountable evidence that Bangladesh, for all its political problems, has come out far ahead of both India and Pakistan in moving towards the minimum development goals as set out by the United Nations and other international agencies. Writing in 2013, economists Jean Drèze and Amartya Sen noted that in the period 1990–2011, as India's per capita income went from being 60 per cent higher than that of Bangladesh to double the income, Bangladesh nevertheless overtook India 'in terms of a wide range of basic social indicators, including life expectancy, child survival, enhanced immunisation rates, reduced fertility rates, and even some (not all) schooling indicators.' It is not accidental that, in comparison with India and Pakistan, Bangladesh has fared far better in mitigating the transmission of the virus and keeping the pandemic-related mortality rate down to one of the lowest in the world.

To some extent, then, there is a case to be made for the argument that countries such as the US and India, which have forgone investments in public health, embraced private healthcare, and therefore left the less affluent and poor to devise their own solutions to healthcare, are now suffering the most due to the coronavirus pandemic. The failure of neoliberal policies in India and Brazil, the drastic consequences of cuts in corporate taxes in all countries, the evisceration of the idea of the commons, the unchecked greed which has led to unspeakably obscene levels of the concentration of wealth in a few hands – all this is a tangible demonstration of what capitalism has wrought. A certain portion of the left in both countries, and of course elsewhere, will be bolder in pronouncing the present crisis as another sign of the imminent collapse of capitalism; some among them will use a heftier language, speaking of the 'structural' flaws in capitalism and the global dynamics that will begin to impede capital accumulation, and thus the faint indicators that now point to the birth of a 'new communism'. We have heard such oracular announcements from time to time, most recently in the aftermath of the 11 September 2001 attacks and during the 2008 financial meltdown, and the more optimistic-minded among the critics of capitalism, who have authored an untold number of articles and books on 'capitalism in crisis', have been heartened by polls suggesting that most young Americans no longer wish to announce themselves to others as 'capitalists'. A Harvard Institute of Politics poll in 2016, for instance, found that only 19 per cent of Americans between ages nineteen and twenty-eight identified themselves as 'capitalists' and 42 per cent said they even 'supported capitalism'. Meanwhile, as the lockdown kept most Americans at home from mid-March to mid-May and sometimes beyond, the Democratic Socialists of America have been gaining new adherents – by the thousands – according to an article in *The Atlantic*. Little do pollsters, or those being polled, know that the 'bitch goddess SUCCESS' has even colonised the dreams of Americans.

The argument, on the other side, has an equally long lineage and the advantage of not having to muster support in grandiose language since America is its living instantiation. Capitalism can withstand shocks, indeed it is so structured as to absorb and even invite them, and every 'crisis' only has the effect of strengthening the ship of capitalism better as its captains learn to navigate their way around the shoals and eddies of turbulence. However rocky the journey, say the adherents of this view, the ship always lands – even if some do not survive the passage, and others must be treated for sickness. Capitalism, on this view, which verges on a form of utilitarianism, is more conducive to the greater happiness of a greater number than any other competing economic systems in the modern world. It is, however, not altogether necessary to anchor oneself firmly in one ideological school or another to arrive at some understanding of what precipitated the onset of Covid-19 itself. If we accept, as there is every reason to do so, what is thus far the most established view, namely that the coronavirus is of zoonotic origins, having originated most likely in bats and perhaps having an intermediate animal reservoir before jumping species and infecting humans, then the question is what this tells us about the political economy that shapes the modern world. There is little doubt that SARS-CoV-2, following the path of HIV, SARS-CoV-1 (2002), H1N1 (Swine Flu, 2009), MERS (2012), and H5N1 (Avian Flu, 2014), is yet another symptom of a trend of highly infectious diseases that appear to be striking the human world. As economies have grown, and as we become increasingly settled into acquisitive societies, humans have ventured further into the wilderness, into habitats that are the reservoirs of pathogens over which we have no control, which we scarcely understand, and which have resented our intrusion. These pathogens are now circulating in our economies.

Viral capitalism has finally met its match in the viral pandemic.

This article was first published as Chapter XI of *The Fury of Covid-19: The Politics, Histories, and Unrequited Love of the Coronavirus* (Pan Macmillan, New Delhi, 2020).

MONTAGU AND OTTOMAN INOCULATION

Iftikhar Malik

> Upon the whole, I look upon the Turkish women as the only free people in the empire.
>
> Montagu to Lady Mar, 1 April 1717

> I allow you to laugh at me for the sensual declaration that I had rather be a rich *effendi* with all his ignorance than Sir Isaac Newton with all his knowledge.
>
> Montagu to Abbe Conti, Constantinople, 19 May 1718.

Historical narratives, like the imperial chronicles, have been dominated by men where either women remain absent, or appear in marginal references unless they are the subject matter themselves and seemingly liable to objectification. In their own times, several women had been travelling to distant lands though, proportionately, left fewer writings for posterity. Amongst some notable names we read about include known queens and scholars such as Queen Sheba of Yemen/Ethiopia (tenth century BC), Queen Cleopatra (69–30 BC), Rabia Basri (731–801), Fatima al-Fihri (800–880) Gulbadan Begum (1523–1603) and Nawab Sikandar Jahan Begum (1817–1868). Colonialism enabled a fair number of European women to visit and write about non-European communities. In cases of the Ottomans, Safawids, Mughals, East Asians and Africans these literary, religious and biographical writings offer ample evidence of interaction across the cultural boundaries. Women like Gertrude Bell (1868–1926), who explored and mapped Syria and Mesopotamia, Freya Stark (1893–1993), who travelled within the Muslim World and wrote about the

Middle East and Afghanistan, and Alexandrine Tinne (1835–1869), who was the first European woman to cross the Sahara, socialised with Muslims in their own ways playing vital roles in contemporary developments while stipulating a multi-layered bonhomie.

Lady Mary Wortley Montagu (1689–1762), English writer and poet, is amongst the earliest European women to engage with Muslims. Her travels across the three continents, encounters with the Turks in the Balkans, Adrianople, Constantinople and further south contextualise her mostly positive views of Muslims. She was born in Holme Pierrepont Hall in Nottinghamshire soon after the English Civil War, the Great Fire of London and the widespread fatalities caused by the plague, particularly in London. The first child of Evelyn Pierrepont, the Duke of Hull-Upon-Kingston, (d. 1726) who was to become Lord Dorchester, and Mary Fielding (d. 1692), Mary Montagu was the eldest among three siblings raised by her paternal grandmother until she was nine. Following her mother's death, when she was just four, Mary spent the next few years in Wiltshire with her grandmother and compensated for her unhappiness there by reading avariciously. Taken into her father's care and not enamoured of her governess, she turned to learning Latin and writing poetry – largely male domains – and by 1695 had already written a short novel and two collections of poetry. Moving between Wiltshire and Nottinghamshire, Montagu refused to marry Clotworthy Skeffington, her father's choice for a suitor, and instead opted for eloping with Edward Wortley Montagu and married this aristocrat-entrepreneur in 1712 in Salisbury. In 1713, Montagu gave birth to a son, moved to London, and soon became a socialite known for her beauty, sense of independence, literary genius and sociability. Her circles included King George I, the Hanoverian king of England, Lady Walpole, Lord and Lady Hervey, Sarah Churchill, the Duchess of Marlborough, Mary Astell, John Gay, Abbe Antonio Conti and Alexander Pope. In 1715, Mary Montagu contracted smallpox but survived, though the epidemic did leave its scars without diminishing her physical charms, self-confidence and social mobility. The following year, her husband was appointed as the British Ambassador to Constantinople and she accompanied him to the Near East passing through the Netherlands, Germany, Austria, Hungary and Serbia before reaching Adrianople and then the Ottoman metropolis. While still in

Constantinople, she gave birth to a daughter in January 1718 and returned to London later in the year, following the inoculation of her son.

She is the first Englishwoman with experience of living in a Muslim society and writing about it while applying her literary skills. Anita Desai considers these few months of her life to be quite special: 'It is highly ironic that out of her long and colourful life, the years best known are the ones she recorded in the *Embassy Letters,* written over a brief period that was lived in foreign parts, far removed from the society and milieu of which she was such a brilliant and celebrated representative.'

Mary Montagu is best known for her letters. As the wife of the British ambassador she had the rare experience of working with higher echelons of the Ottoman sultanate and might have been the only Westerner to have a close relationship with the royal family besides interacting with elite Ottoman women – otherwise an inaccessible area for Western men. It is largely owing to these direct encounters during an era of recurrent pestilences, such as smallpox, that she tried to espouse the case for inoculation back in Britain. She challenged the long-held taboos on domesticity and conformity; and has left us five volumes of extensive writings with her letters in particular covering a wide range of topics other than her first-hand reportage on the Ottoman culture. A self-confident person, Montagu survived smallpox, which, for a while, left its scars on her face, yet refused to circumvent her public profile and creative pursuits. Her independent-mindedness, evident from her relationship with Alexander Pope, Lord Hervey and Abbe Conti, would not allow her to make compromises expected of women of her times. Her wedding with Edward Wortley Montagu – the scion of a moneyed family – was not a love marriage but was partly meant to escape an arranged matrimony, which was the norm in contemporary English upper classes. Not enamoured of such arrangements, she noted: 'People in my way are sold like slaves: and I cannot tell what price my master will put on me'. Her brother, William, was also forced to marry while quite young to a teenage Rachel Baynton. Following his death at twenty of smallpox, his eighteen-year-old widow had to look after their two children. Montagu had prophesied this mismatch and was determined not to undergo a similar fate. In England, considerations such as pedigree, land, money and dowry often determined match making, where women, in particular, did not enjoy much choice with the decisions often left to fathers. In contrast, Montagu found Ottoman women, unlike the usual stereotypes, more independent, and despite the veil or such homebound roles, they often maintained their own autonomy in several matters.

Montagu corresponded with her male friends during her marriage without hiding her relationship or glossing over it; instead, she later chose to live in France and Italy pursuing an independent life, not much in vogue during that period. Some admiring men, including Alexander Pope, felt unreciprocated by Montagu and turned quite hostile in their writings, though she would not allow false expectations unless she herself felt a modicum of intimacy. As borne out by her letters to Pope, she liked and respected the poet but never let him entertain any special romantic attachment though the former felt a bitter sense of betrayal. She was appreciative of his mentoring and it was on his persuasion that her familiar portrait in an Ottoman dress was commissioned but then she knew eminent intellectuals such as Voltaire, Joseph Addison, Richard Steele and William Congrave who, in their own ways, acknowledged her credentials as an independent and creative soul. Montagu had her due share of idiosyncrasies, and often bluntly blurted out her opinions, which might have bordered on sheer arrogance, or even racism. For instance, during her visit to Carthage, she wrote disparaging remarks about African women and described her own granddaughter as ugly. Her observations about Austrian women were equally harsh as were the remarks about profligacy among their German counterparts. At one stage, she had advocated the abolition of parliament with all the powers returning to a sovereign king.

Mary Montagu's convoy, including the provisions of twenty liveries, a chaplain and other paraphernalia, took off for the Continent in August 1716, preferring to take a land route to firm up relations with the Austrian monarchy. In Vienna, a triumphalist ambience prevailed following Prince Eugene's decisive victory over the Ottomans at Peterwardein (Novi Sad) in July 1716. The Ottoman troops, led by the Grand Vizier, Damat Ali, had been defeated by a combination of Austrian, Serb, Hungarian, Croat and Venetian soldiers who fought under the banner of the Holy Roman Empire. Only 50,000 Janissaries, Sepoys and Tartars from the 120,000-strong army escaped the battlefield by the Danube while Damat Ali was himself killed in action, thus making this battle a turning point for

Osmanlis led by Sultan Ahmed III (1673–1730). The late Grand Vizier was an important member of the royal family since he had married Fatima, one of the several daughters of the Ottoman Sultan. Lady Montagu was to meet Fatima subsequently in Adrianople and was quite taken in by her beauty, wisdom and resolution. The Wortleys witnessed extensive celebrations in Vienna given their two-month stay and partying in the capital before they took off for Belgrade via Prague, Dresden and Leipzig. In Budapest, she witnessed the scars from the recent battles besides the ongoing civil war between the Catholics and Protestants until they travelled through Serbia, where, unlike Austria and Hungary, she noticed widespread poverty. She personally witnessed the battleground of Peterwardein where 30,000 Turkish dead had been Janissaries, and many other Sepoys had been taken as prisoners. In her letter to Alexander Pope from Belgrade on 12 February 1717, she noted: 'No attempt was made to bury the dead....The marks of that Glorious bloody day are yet recent, the field being stew'd with the Skulls and Carcases of unbury'd Men, Horses and Camels. I could not look without horror on such numbers of mangled humane bodys, and reflect on the Injustice of War, that makes murther not only necessary but meritorious'.

Encounters with the Ottomans

Mary Montagu's memorable encounter of civilisational nature with a Muslim Turk happened in Belgrade where the Wortleys stayed in the private residence of Achmed Bey who also housed their large ambassadorial guard for several weeks. More like a count, as she wrote to Pope, Bey's father had been a senior official who ensured for his son

> the most polite eastern learning, being perfectly skilled in Arabic and Persian languages, and is an extraordinary scribe, which they call *effendi*. This accomplishment makes way to the greatest preferments, but he has had the good sense to prefer an easy, quiet, secure life to all the dangerous honour of the Porte. He sups with us every night, and drinks wine very freely. You cannot imagine how much he is delighted with the liberty of conversing with me. He has explained to me many pieces of the Arabian poetry which, I observed, are in numbers not unlike ours, generally alternate verse, and of a very musical sound. Their expressions of love are very passionate and lively.

It appears that Achmed Bey was discussing ghazal, the genre of romantic poetry where each couplet is rhymed with the preceding one and self-sufficient in its contents very unlike the normative poem. Continuing in her letter to the English poet, Montagu further noted:

> I am so much pleased with them, I really believe I should learn to read Arabic, if I was to stay here a few months. He has a very good library of their books of all kinds and, as he tells me, spends the greatest part of his life there. I pass for a great scholar with him, by relating to him some of the Persian tales, which I find are genuine. At first he believed I understood Persian. I have frequent disputes with him concerning the differences of our customs, particularly the confinements of women. He assures me, there is nothing at all in it; only, says he, we have the advantage when our wives cheat us nobody knows. He has wit, and is more polite than many Christian men of quality.

Lady Montagu's proverbial big moment arrived when she went to visit the household of the Grand Vizier, accompanied by two ladies, a guide and a Greek translator, followed by a spontaneous visit to another household where her host, Fatima, made a lasting mark on her. Without mentioning her royal genealogy, Montagu waxes lyrical of Fatima's beauty as it further underlines her views about the Ottoman women and their health - away from the usual representations of oppressed weaklings. Once settled in Pera, she adorned the Turkish *yasmak* (veil) which helped the English ambassadress in her mobility in bazaars, mosques, shrines and other places of cultural interest. While wearing Ottoman costume, she even ventured to see Aya Sofia though she had to seek prior permission to visit the premises given its history as well as sensitivity. She was quite impressed by its dome of 113-foot diameter, built on arches and supported by gigantic marble pillars, whereas the inner space featured two galleries along with the resting place of the Emperor Constantine. She thought Suleiman's Mosque was the perfect symbol of architectural synthesis and aesthetics and believed Valide Mosque to be the largest among all the mosques in the city, which made her proud as it was commissioned by a woman – the mother of Sultan Mohammed IV. In her letter to Lady Bristol on this preeminent mosque, Montagu opined: 'Between friends, St Paul's Church would make a pitiful figure near it, as any of our squares would be near the Atmeydan, or Place of Horses'. She was all praise for Sultan Achmed's Mosque and accused some Greeks for sharing negative views with other Westerners in the City.

She also visited some *hans* and monasteries which did not impress her given their ordinariness. In one case, she visited a monastery *(tekke)* to see the whirling dervishes. In the same letter to Lady Bristol, she described the various rituals unique to the dervishes—all the way from their plain clothes, conical hats to body movements that began with the Qur'anic recitation by their leader to shift into rhythmic dance:

> The whole is performed with the most solemn gravity. Nothing can be more austere than the form of these people. They never raise their eyes and seem devoted to contemplations, and as ridiculous as this is in description there is something touching in the air of submission and mortification they assume.

In a similar letter to Abbe Conti, the Venetian scholar and a friend of Isaac Newton, Montagu offered extensive details, among other subjects, on the architectural aspects of the Ottoman mosques. She provided interesting searchlight on Sultan Selim's Mosque in Adrianople, a marvel created by the famous architect, Mimar Senan (1489–1588), himself buried near Sulemaniya Mosque and Tombs in Istanbul. She visited the mosque in her Turkish habit and was 'officiously' well received by the caretaker who took her around to see the premises. Passing through the first court with four doors and the innermost with three, she saw herself 'surrounded with cloisters with the marble pillars of the Ionic order, finely polished and of very lively colours, the whole pavement being white marble'. She noticed the roof built in the design of a large dome with several cupolas, and the four marble fountains for decorative purposes. Marvelling at the immensely high dome, she found it to be the 'noblest building I ever saw'. She noticed two rows of marble galleries anchored on pillars and balustrades with the main floor covered by Persian carpets. She felt these details more enticing than the Catholic churches with their 'tawdry images and pictures' and looking like 'toyshops'. One wonders whether these observations about Catholic churches are out of exuberance, or a considered opinion by an Anglican! She wondered about the glazed walls, and on a closer examination found the veneer to be made of 'japan china', though in fact, these are well-known Iznik ceramic tiles. Behind the mosque, she noticed a charity centre housing several dervishes whose simple attires and conical woollen hats gave them a unique appearance. She found them absorbed in their rituals but offered no further details. They might have been whirling dervishes from the Mvelvi order of Maulana Rumi of Konya, or disciples of some other Sufi order.

Montagu's views are in sharp contrast to the then prevailing view of the Ottoman empire in England, best represented in *The General Historie of the Turkes* (1603) by Richard Knolles. It is considered the earliest work in English on the Ottomans. Knolles, highlighting the contemporary Christian view of world history, sought a divine scheme behind the rise of the Turks. Unlike the past Latin works, this pioneer English volume showed Turks as superstitious infidels, who were able to exploit the weaknesses of the contemporary Christians. It underwent several printings and left its enduring imprints on parallel images of the Ottomans, rooted in the Renaissance era.

Ambassador Wortley was recalled to London after completing only a year in Constantinople largely because of his sympathetic attitude towards Ottoman stance vis-à-vis the Austrians and because of subversive nuances of the British Ambassador in Vienna, Abraham Stanyan. Stanyan conspired to have Wortley removed and successfully convinced the foreign office that Wortley's terms for peace between Constantinople and Vienna were unacceptable. The Admiralty deputed a ship to bring the Wortleys back and thus ended this sojourn rather too quickly with Montagu feeling quite mellow. In January 1718, she gave birth to a girl while on 18 March, their four-year old son, Edward Wortley Montagu was inoculated in Constantinople. The journey back home began on 6 June 1718. By that time, Montagu had already learnt the language and knew several members and families from amongst the Ottoman elite, as she noted in a letter to Conti in May of the same year: 'I have not been yet a full year here and am on the point of removing; such is my rambling destiny. This will surprise you, and can surprise anybody so much as myself.' The Wortleys, now four in number, left Constantinople on *The Preston* and while passing through the Dardanelles, visited historic sites such as Abydos, Sigeum, Kadikoy and Troy.

It was from here that Montagu sent an exhaustive letter to Conti commenting on the historical places well known in Homer's writings besides their linkages with the Perso-Greek wars in the ancient era. Given Conti's interest in classics and Montagu's own penchant for Greek mythology, she visited the promontory of Sigeum, where as per mythological narratives, Achilles had been buried 'and where Alexander ran naked round his tomb in his honour'. Ambassador Wortley picked up a marble slab from the site, which on his return, he donated to Trinity College, his alma mater in Cambridge, where it presently lodges in the entrance. Following a voyage around Sicily and a short visit to a heavily fortified Malta, their ship landed at Tunis, where the local British consul, Richard Lawrence, took a curious Montagu on a nocturnal visit of the ruins of Carthage. It was a Ramadan night with a full moon and Montagu was enchanted by the spectacle especially when she, like local people, munched on melons, figs and dates. She returned from her exploratory tour only at daybreak and did not seem to like the treeless vistas featuring a sandy desert and her encounters with the natives. In the letter to the Venetian intellectual, while describing the features of the local inhabitants, she bordered on sheer racism: 'We saw under the trees in many places companies of the country people eating, singing and dancing to their wild music. They are not quite black, but all mulattoes, and the most frightful creatures they can appear in a human figure'. During the day, she saw some urban women who, despite covered in veil from head to toe, were 'mixed with a breed of renegades, are said to be ... fair and handsome'. However, when she went out to see some more Roman ruins now used as granaries, a few peasant women flocked to see her: 'Their posture in sitting, the colour of their skin, their lank black hair falling on each side their faces, their features and the shape of their limbs differ so little from their own country people, the baboons, 'tis hard to fancy them a distinct race, and I could not help thinking here had been some ancient alliances between them'.

Ottoman Inoculation

During Montagu's lifetime, two epidemics, plague and smallpox, were prevalent. Almost every community suffered with millions losing their lives. Called 'the speckled monster', smallpox was the deadliest on earth, eventually claiming more people than the Black Death. One in four infected persons would die with the rest inflicted with life-long and deep-pitted scars. Montagu herself had been a sufferer of smallpox and, as mentioned earlier, lost her twenty-year-old brother to the virus. Like plague, smallpox was a periodic visitor, and generated considerable discussion about possible treatment or preventive cures.

While residing in Constantinople, Montagu had been asked about these pandemics and their hazards for visitors like her and, given the specific images about the Ottomans, some of her friends worried about her health. As she explained in a letter written in April 1718 to Sarah Chiswell, a few neighbours and even their own cook in Adrianople caught smallpox but Montagu did not know it until after their recovery. She thought that the Ottoman people took plague in their own stride but to ward off smallpox they depended on inoculation conducted by traditional women mendicants. She saw many people escaping death since grafting smallpox infection into their veins would successfully trigger a stronger response from the immune system disallowing infection to germinate itself. While reassuring Chiswell of her own safety and of some other Europeans under the English protection, she informed her of such an operation and its healing properties:

> The smallpox, so fatal and so general amongst us, is here entirely harmless by the invention of engrafting, which is the term they give it. There is a set of old women who make it their business to perform the operation. Every autumn in the month of September when the great heat is abated, people send one another to know if any of their family has a mind to have the smallpox. They make parties for this purpose and when they are met (commonly fifteen or sixteen together) the old woman comes with nutshell full of the matter of the best sort of smallpox, and asks what veins you please to have opened. She immediately rips open that you offer to her with a large needle (which gives you no more pain than a common scratch) and puts into the vein as much venom as can lie upon the head of her needle, and after binds up the little wound with a hollow bit of shell, and in this manner opens four or five veins.

According to Montagu, the Greeks usually preferred to have grafts on their foreheads in the shape of a cross but would often end up with lifetime scars whereas other people would have them on legs or arms. Following this operation, everybody will go back to their normal routine until a week later when they would catch fever keeping them bedridden for a few days. Their recovery happened quickly though the cuts on their bodies would take time to heal and there was reportedly

> no example of any one that has died in it, and you may believe I am well satisfied of the safety of the experiment, since I intend to try it on my dear little son. I am patriot enough to take pains to bring this useful invention into fashion in England and I should not fail to write to some of our doctors very particularly about it if I knew anyone of them that I thought had virtue enough to destroy such a considerable branch of their revenue for the good of mankind.

However, she was not hopeful of support for inoculation back in England. In letters to her husband, while he was in Adrianople paying his farewell visit to the Court, Montagu informed him of their son's inoculation on 18 March 1718, and speedy recovery. On 23 March, she told her spouse of the younger Montagu 'at this time singing and playing and very impatient for supper … I cannot engraft the girl: her nurse has not had the smallpox'. Following this rather brief letter giving more space to financial matters than to children's health, Montagu wrote another to her husband a week later, which ironically, had only a single opening line on their son, as she noted: 'Your son is as well as can be expected, and I hope past all manner of danger'. Given the nature of their marital relationship, the letters read drily and are formulated in a rather impersonal way. Even a major family matter such as the inoculation of their son or reference to their newly-born daughter is quite cursory.

On her return to England, Montagu tried to persuade her social circles and royalty on following the Ottoman practice, at least among the younger people, but faced fierce resistance including rebukes from priests and scientists. But she never gave up. Her Italian friend, Conti, had already left London but she immersed herself in buying books and writing down her travel experiences, originally reflected in her letters. A smitten Pope encouraged Montagu in her literary pursuits besides commissioning Godfrey Kneller to make her portrait wearing a modified Turkish habit in London. Amidst growing estrangement with Pope leading to more acrimonious outbursts from the poet, Montagu became intensely engaged in the contemporary debate on smallpox already polarised between those who advocated prevention versus those who focused on its treatment. In an unusual warm winter of 1721, epidemic returned to England with the fear of contagion totally freezing socialisation amongst the upper classes. Montagu asked Charles Maitland, the former embassy doctor now working in Hereford, to inoculate her daughter. Given the contemporary criticism, he involved three other physicians in the process and, until younger Mary's total recovery, several people kept visiting her. Maitland's successful procedures in front of his critical colleagues were enough to persuade several other opinion makers though it was difficult to convince the royal family. Caroline, the Princess of Wales, supported Montagu. But her father-in-law, King George I, asked for a prior experimental testing on some proverbial guinea pigs. Accordingly, six inmates – three men and three women – from Newgate prison were engrafted with infected fluids and within a few days, all of them felt normal. The King was still not satisfied and would not allow his grandchildren to be inoculated. So another experiment on eleven orphans took place with similar positive results. Consequently, Princess Caroline's daughters were inoculated on 17 April 1721, making the practice more acceptable within the society though the controversy in print media continued for some time with Mary Montagu contributing pieces under a pseudonym. It was a generation later that Edward Jenner (1749–1823) familiarised the method of injecting cowpox instead of more dangerous smallpox into the human body – a process that came to be known as vaccination.

Like many of her contemporaries, Mary Montagu personified some idiosyncrasies of her times and class, yet the fact remains that her innovative ideas, her defiant views about the Ottoman societies, especially their women, literary and cultural aesthetics and certainly the Ottoman way of preventing smallpox, earned her a unique position, which went against the given norms of the time. Her untraditional life style, relationship with literary figures while keeping her own autonomy and her role in accepting and advocating inoculation put her centuries ahead of her time. As a symbol of several Enlightenment ideas, she saw Muslim society without any preordained biases, irreverent to praise or fear. Montagu stood prominently in her own league as a feminist whose inspirations grew from a substantial and unique encounter with Muslim society.

COVID-19, ISLAM AND PSEUDOSCIENCE

Nidhal Guessoum

The coronavirus pandemic has affected millions of lives and wrecked large parts of humanity's life, from economic activity to sports, including education and religious life. Who will forget seeing the haram in Mecca (the space around the Kaaba) empty for weeks or months, and Pope Francis delivering Easter mass from an empty basilica or, days earlier, giving *Urbi et Orbi* (to the city and the world) blessing in an empty St Peter's Square.

All religions of the world have been tested in various and unprecedented ways by this crisis. A number of questions have been raised. Is this pandemic an act of God, some test or punishment? Should believers rely on medicine and science or just pray and trust in their faiths? Will God intervene and somehow get rid of the pandemic if many devout people offer heartfelt prayers? Will religious activities (sermons, collective prayers, etc.) evolve in response to the new circumstances or will tradition prove more sturdy? Will this crisis bring people back to religion (if they conclude that the pandemic was because they had angered God), or will it drive many away (if they cannot understand why God let this suffering happen – to even the nicest of us)? How will science and religion interact during and after this pandemic crisis – will rationality make progress or will irrationality find fertile ground to flourish anew?

These are all important questions that not only apply to all religions but also interest all people, religious or not. They are new examples of the eternal debates between religion, reason and science. How does one approach the above questions: from the religious angle or from the rational, scientific side? And how does one determine what is essential and what is just habitual in religious beliefs and practices?

In the Islamic world, however, in addition to the above questions being raised and addressed – albeit not nearly with the attention they deserve

– large sections of society have reacted in surprising and rather worrisome ways.

First, in the early phase of the pandemic, a theologically primitive attitude was expressed, viewing and presenting the pandemic as a divine punishment, or even revenge, against China (more on this below). Then, when the pandemic hit the rest of the world, including Muslim peoples, the attitude changed into an appropriation, claiming that it was announced in the Qur'an and that the Prophet had told Muslims and the world what measures should be adopted in such situations – preceding science and its procedures. Interestingly, in attempting to prove that many Islamic acts and rituals do constitute hygienic and scientifically supported actions that help in the prevention, slow down, and treatment of Covid-19, many Muslim writers often replaced science with pseudoscience.

The (still unfolding) story of Covid-19 and Islam thus presents an interesting topic of study of three important subjects: theology, *i`jaz* (the famous 'miraculous scientific contents in the Qur'an and the Sunna, the Prophetic Tradition'), and pseudoscience.

Covid-19 and Islamic Theology

On the theological level, how is one to think of the pandemic? What is God's role and place in all this? What roles do reason and 'pure faith' play in thinking about this?

To address these questions and others, the Yaqeen Institute for Islamic Research surveyed over 1,800 practising American Muslims of diverse profiles (age, education, and ethnicity). To the question 'Is the coronavirus a punishment from Allah?', the respondents were equally split between 'No' ('Not at all' or 'A little') and 'Yes' ('A moderate amount', 'A lot', or 'A great deal'). And to the question 'Is the coronavirus a test from Allah?', 84 per cent said that it is a *major* test from Allah.

The authors of the Yaqeen Institute paper then offered commentary on the results and the related issues. They cited hadiths from Prophet Muhammad that declare plague-like epidemics and other such afflictions as earthly punishments from Allah. These are supposed to serve as reminders of God's power and bring us back to Him in order to avoid 'greater punishments' in the hereafter. However, the paper insisted that 'it is beyond human perception' to know the exact causes behind such 'nearer punishments', or who (if any people in particular) they are directed to. The paper added that this divine act can even be a blessing 'for the believer who exercises patience, appropriately quarantines him or herself, hopes in reward from Allah, and accepts that whatever happens is from Allah's divine decree.' But if one cannot make sense of such an act (why and against whom), how can one digest it? The perplexity and doubts remain unresolved.

The Islamic popular and pseudo-scholarly discourse, however, was even more troubling.

When the virus first appeared in China, and the Chinese government took drastic lockdown measures, some conservative Islamic personalities, websites, YouTube channels, and Facebook pages, claimed that the coronavirus was 'revenge from God', as the Chinese had locked nearly a million Muslims from the Uighur minority of the Xinjiang region in concentration camps. The punishment, it was stressed, was of the same kind as the crime (locking down millions of people), which confirms that it is a retribution. Some preachers went so far as saying that developing a cure to the disease could be an attempt to resist God's will! One important Islamic personality who promoted and defended this view is Ahmad Issa Al-Maasarawy, Professor of Hadith at Al-Azhar University, chairman of the Committee for the Recitation of the Qur'an, and former Sheikh of the Egyptian Diar (religious institution), who has over 930,000 followers on Twitter. On 26 January 2020, he tweeted: 'After China isolated more than 5 million Uighurs, today the whole world is isolating China because of the spread of the deadly corona pandemic among the Chinese and the fear of spreading the infection. (And your Lord is not unjust toward people (Qur'an 41:46)).' His tweet received 14,500 likes, 5,100 retweets, and 555 replies.

Additional Qur'anic verses and Prophetic statements were quoted as arguments in support of such views and reasoning:

- And who does more oppression than those who forbid that Allah's Name be glorified and mentioned in His mosques and strive for their ruin? It was not fitting that such should enter them (Allah's Mosques) except in fear. For them there is disgrace in this world, and they will have a great torment in the Hereafter. (Qur'an 2:114)

- So each We punished for his sin. Some of them were struck by a violent sand-storm, some by a blast of sound, others were swallowed up by the earth, and some were drowned (in the sea). God did not do injustice to them, but they had wronged themselves. (Qur'an 29:40)
- And no one knows the soldiers of your Lord except Him. (Qur'an 74:31)
- A hadith narrated by Bukhari states: On the authority of Aisha, May Allah be pleased with her, she said: I asked the Messenger of God (Peace Be Upon Him) about the plague, and he told me that its torment inflicted by Allah on whomever He wills, and that Allah has made it a mercy for the believers: anyone who gets hit by the plague but stays in his country with patience and forbearance, knowing that he will only suffer what Allah has decreed to him, he will receive the same reward as a martyr (even if he doesn't die).

Another Islamic personality who promoted this retribution standpoint is Mohamed Elzoghbe, a controversial Egyptian preacher, who in an episode on the YouTube channel Al-Rahma (which has over 100,000 subscribers) stated: 'Yesterday, China isolated a million Muslims and is still isolating them, and today it isolates 18 million Chinese and is still isolating them. Indeed, the penalty is of the same kind as the act. If the enemy looks at Muslims, and the [lack of] strength of Muslims and flouts it, know that it is then God, the Higher Authority, who intervenes.'

When the virus reached Muslim populations and countries, the Islamic (popular) discourse shifted from presenting the virus that 'descended as a soldier of God to retaliate against the oppressing Chinese' to describing it as a test for the believers, aiming to determine who will show patience with this affliction and who will be resentful. Preachers called on the faithful to redouble on prayers and supplications, to ask Allah to take away the scourge.

Moderate voices tried to balance prayer and science and recalled the famous advice that the Prophet gave to a Bedouin who wondered whether he should tie his camel or rely on God: 'tie it… and trust in God' was the reply.

Similarly, others tried to find 'scientific' arguments within the Islamic tradition. Many thus recalled the Prophet's recommendations on hygiene, generally, and behaviour during epidemics, in particular. People cited hadiths in which the Prophet instructed Muslims to avoid places where an epidemic has appeared, or to remain and not leave the place if one is already there, to separate the sick from the healthy, to regard cleanliness as part of faith, and to seek medical treatment for any illness. Many declared the Prophet as prescient, even reading 'social distancing' in some of his statements.

Indeed, this pandemic reignited the debates of reason and faith: how to think of such events and how to act in consequence.

Covid and I`jaz

I`jaz is the widespread claim that various scientific discoveries, whether natural or cosmic phenomena or scientific explanations and theories, have been mentioned in the Qur'an or in the Prophet's Sunna (statements, acts, directives), preceding and anticipating scientific developments by over a thousand years and thus constituting proof of the Qur'an's divine origin and of Muhammad's prophethood. I`jaz is often translated as 'scientific miracles in the Qur'an and the Sunna'; I prefer the slightly different expression 'scientific miraculous content in the Qur'an and the Sunna'. It is extremely popular in contemporary Muslim culture, with countless books, videos, TV programs, websites, encyclopedias, conferences, and dedicated 'scholarly' societies such as the International Commission for Scientific Miracles (or Miraculous Content) of the Qur'an and Sunnah, symbolically established in Mecca under the auspices of the World Muslim League.

The I`jaz phenomenon has been studied, criticised and debunked at some length by a string of scholars. Critiques have also started to appear in Arabic, in both scholarly works and popular presentations. However, the popularity of this phenomenon has not declined. On the contrary, the Covid-19 crisis seems to have given it a boost.

A video posted on 31 January 2020 was titled 'God Almighty informed us about the coronavirus, and the Messenger, Peace Be Upon Him, informed us about the secret of its treatment'; within a few weeks, it was watched over 20 million times and it received close to half a million likes, with a 96 per cent like ratio. In a post that went viral on Facebook, the coronavirus was declared as having been mentioned in the Qur'an, more specifically in Chapter 74. Verses 11 to 13 read: 'Leave Me [to deal] with him whom I created lonely, and whom I have granted abundant wealth, and children present [with him]', while verses 26 to 30 read: 'I will cast him into hell. Would that you really knew what hell is! It leaves and spares no one and nothing. It scorches people's skin/flesh. Over it are nineteen.' First, the 'abundant wealth and children present' in the passage above are claimed to refer to China, and the number nineteen is linked to Covid-19, even though it has always been understood as referring to the number of angels who guard over hell. Finally, the term 'corona' is decried because it has 'obviously' been extracted from Coran/Koran/Qur'an!

Such pronouncements made the rounds of social media so quickly and widely that the Egyptian Authority for Fatwas felt obliged to post a statement on its Facebook page declaring that the alleged mention of the coronavirus in the Qur'an is 'a slander and a lie'. The Authority described this claim as 'misrepresenting the Qur'an and distorting the meaning of God's verses,' insisting that 'we believe that God Almighty has commanded us to use causal relations while trusting in Him and praying to Him; indeed, the remedy for this [outbreak] is to follow the health instructions from the Ministry of Health and praying to God Almighty to lift the epidemic, not in spreading myths and trying to prove something that has no truth.'

Abd Al-Daim Al-Kaheel, who has specialised in I`jaz and has an 'encyclopedia' online on the subject, wrote the following in an article on his website (undated, but posted sometime in March or April 2020): 'I could not have imagined reading an article about the scientific miraculousness of the Sunnah in a western newspaper and by an American professor, Craig Considine, a professor of sociology at Rice University.' He was referring to an op-ed by Considine in *Newsweek* titled 'Can the Power of Prayer Alone Stop a Pandemic like the Coronavirus? Even the Prophet Muhammad Thought Otherwise'. Al-Kaheel quoted Considine referring to the Prophet's directives to people to avoid going into or leaving towns where the plague has appeared and 'to adhere to hygienic practices'. Al-Kaheel then concluded: 'We now say: Have people in the West begun to realise the importance of the teachings of Islam in preventing epidemics? Actually, who told Muhammad, may God's prayers and peace be upon him, about these facts, which physicians did not realise until after the epidemic spread?'

This is typical of the I`jazi discourse: a rush to exaggerate statements made by Westerners that seem to support Islamic ideas or practices conflating valid practices (in this case hygienic or health-related) with historic and scientific precedence, and oftentimes misrepresenting and/or misunderstanding someone's actual thesis. Indeed, Al-Kaheel and the countless others who shared and disseminated Considine's article online do not seem to have realised that the author was making a different point: that even the great prophet of Islam did not advocate prayer as a way to react to or counter an epidemic, but rather instructed his followers to adhere to known socio-medical rules.

The key word in the previous sentence is 'known', for indeed what the Prophet was advocating was known in the medicine of his times. Here is what Ibn Khaldun, the great historian and sociologist of the fourteenth century, wrote in the section on medicine of his magnum opus *Introduction to History*:

> The medicine mentioned in religious tradition is of the (Bedouin) type. It is in no way part of the divine revelation. (Such medical matters) were merely (part of) Arab custom and happened to be mentioned in connection with the circumstances of the Prophet, like other things that were customary in his generation. They were not mentioned in order to imply that that particular way of practising (medicine) is stipulated by the religious law. Muhammad was sent to teach us the religious law. He was not sent to teach us medicine or any other ordinary matter. In connection with the story of the fecundation of the palms, he said: 'You know more about your worldly affairs (than I).'
>
> None of the statements concerning medicine that occur in sound traditions should be considered to (have the force of) law. There is nothing to indicate that this is the case. The only thing is that if that type of medicine is used for the sake of a divine blessing and in true religious faith, it may be very useful.

In the previous paragraph, Ibn Khaldun introduces Bedouin medicine as follows:

> Civilised Bedouins have a kind of medicine which is mainly based upon individual experience. They inherit its use from the *shaykhs* and old women of the tribe. Some of it may occasionally be correct. However, (that kind of medicine) is not based upon any natural norm or upon any conformity (of the treatment) to the temper of the humours. Much of this sort of medicine

existed among the Arabs. They had well-known physicians, such as al-Harith b. Kaladah and others.

In addition to these statements by Ibn Khaldun about the medical knowledge of the time and the non-religious nature of the Prophet's recommendations, one can also refer to poems and oral traditions that mention the plague and the common practice of isolating or 'confining' those struck by it.

Pseudoscientific Claims

Caleb Lack and Jacques Rousseau give a 'common-sense definition' of pseudoscience in their recent book *Critical Thinking, Science, and Pseudoscience:* 'any claim, hypothesis, or theory that is presented in the language and manner typical of scientific claims, but that fails to conform to accepted standards in science regarding openness to peer review, replicability, transparent methodology, and the potential for falsifiability is highly likely to be a pseudoscientific claim, hypothesis, or theory.' Examples of pseudoscientific claims include the insistence that practices such as homeopathy, astrology, cupping and bloodletting, and more, are valid and true and that there is more than enough evidence to justify one's belief in their validity, usefulness, and truth. Lack and Rousseau note that 'it is very easy to find evidence for those claims' and 'any claims made in pseudoscientific discourse can typically not be falsified'. Scott Lillenfeld explains that pseudoscience comprises 'an absence of self-correction, overuse of ad hoc manoeuvres to immunise claims from refutation, use of scientific-sounding but vacuous language, extraordinary claims in the absence of compelling evidence, overreliance on anecdotal and testimonial assertions, avoidance of peer review, and the like'.

A timeline analysis of the term 'pseudoscience' (using Ngram, the Google programme which allows one to analyse the usage and relative prevalence of a term, name or expression in books since 1800) shows that while the term has been in use since at least 1820, its usage suddenly increased around 1970, plateaued roughly between 1980 and 1990, then resumed its exponential increase until today. Historian of science David Hecht explains this emergent interest in pseudoscience: 'the explosion of pseudoscience over the past fifty years is thus a product both of the high status of science and the persistent concerns that nonscientists have frequently harboured about science.'

It is not always obvious to everyone that pseudoscientific beliefs and practices are harmful to people. One often hears: what is the harm in reading horoscopes and assigning some level of truth to them? In the case of homeopathy, will it not at the very least have the benefit of a placebo? As to cupping and bloodletting, people will usually admit that if these practices are not done cleanly enough, there is a risk of infection, of excessive bleeding, or other such ailments, but those who believe in cupping and bloodletting (for anecdotal or 'religious' reasons) will insist that the practitioners perform these actions with utmost care. What remains is the financial cost, and people will argue that modern medicine is often much more costly than these traditional treatments, so the latter's harm is far from established. Those of us who understand science and why modern medicinal treatment can be trusted much more than those traditional methods (because of the rigorous scientific methodology behind testing and approval) know that the real harm of those pseudoscientific practices lies in the fact that they keep the patients from real, effective treatments (leaving aside intellectual pollution and confusion). The typical literature of pseudoscience relies heavily on anecdotes ('I know many people who tried this and it worked for them'), on the argument from authority ('this defender and promoter of bloodletting has a medical degree, many years of practice, and many articles and videos'), the usage of scientific terms or jargon, and cherry-picking of evidence and cases.

When Covid-19 began to spread far and wide, people were reminded that this was not our first encounter with a coronavirus (SARS-CoV-2 in this case). We had previously had MERS-CoV, the Middle Eastern respiratory syndrome disease, which infected about 2,500 people and killed about a thousand since April 2012 when it first appeared in Saudi Arabia. In 2014, the International Commission for Scientific Miracles of the Qur'an and Sunnah, had issued a statement on Islamic ways for the prevention and treatment of the MERS coronavirus disease, ways that it said were derived from the Qur'an and the Sunnah 'under the supervision of [its] Scientific Committee'. The recommendations were a mixture of religious activities (recitations of special prayers and supplications) to 'prevent' infections, and health-related practices that raise the efficiency of one's immune system.

However, as Sheikh Abdullah Al-Musleh, the Secretary General of the Commission, stressed in those statements, some activities, such as ablutions (the washing of hands, face, arms and feet before the formal prayers) could actually be considered as part of both the religious and the health-related acts. Indeed, Al-Musleh recommended increasing water inhalations (while washing one's nose during ablutions), increasing the consumption of honey ('dissolved in a cup of water twice daily'), and eating seven dates ('preferably of the Ajwa kind') each day on an empty stomach. He insisted that these practices were all part of the Prophet's tradition and would help prevent infections. Furthermore, he recommended traditional treatments for the sick: two grams a day of black seed and one small spoon of the saussurea plant in a cup of boiled water, morning and evening. He also noted the importance of physical activity and of a healthy diet, with vegetables, particularly pumpkin and broccoli, fresh fruits, and ginger with tea. And last, but not to be left out, he recommended the usage of bloodletting. In the end, he did stress, however, that a patient should always seek the advice of a medical specialist.

Al-Musleh insisted that these recommendations, while derived from the Qur'an and the Sunnah, are all scientifically documented and in line with current research on the immune system, for the Commission's scientific committee includes, according to him, world-class specialists, and the Commission's scientific conclusions are presented in conferences and published in its Journal of Scientific Miracles. Needless to say, the 'medical'/health/hygiene recommendations of Al-Musleh and the Commission have no scientific support or evidence whatsoever. They are a mixture of centuries-old folk medicine and of pseudo-scientific claims and acts, such as bloodletting.

During the 2020 pandemic, however, Islam-related pseudoscientific claims got even worse.

Professor Johan Giesecke, a Swedish top expert in epidemiology, was quoted as saying (in an interview he gave to Swedish Radio on 22 April 2020): 'I can almost assuredly state that fasting reduces the risk of infection with the coronavirus, because moisture provides the appropriate environment for the incubation of one's mucous membranes, and I believe that the risk of transmission is reduced when fasting.' (I could not verify the accuracy of the statement, as reported, for I unfortunately do not know Swedish.) In the article citing this interview and statement, Al-Kaheel comments: 'But this professor advises fasting people to rinse the mouth several times every day... He also advises doctors to clean exposed parts such as hands, face and nose several times a day... In other words he advises ablution!' Further in the same article, he asks: 'But does fasting help patients? Yale University recently paid attention to fasting, so it conducted a study that was published in 2016 in the journal *Cell*; it found that humans and animals alike when infected with diseases lose their appetite naturally... This is an automatic body reaction and an innate indication of the need to practice fasting during illness... and experience has shown that some diseases are completely cured by just practising fasting!'

This idea of 'moisturising the mouth and nose' through ablutions as a helpful action in preventing coronavirus infections was relayed by others, with the additional claim that it is a recommendation of the World Health Organization. Here we see the usage of pseudoscience in an I`jazi approach. Needless to say, the recommendations of the World Health Organization, on the ways to help prevent infections by the coronavirus, not only do not make such claims, but rather only stress that washing the nose with saline solutions does not prevent coronavirus infections.

Another claim connected beards to the protection from the coronavirus. In an interview with the online news site Sotaliraq.com (The Voice of Iraq), Osama Saad Al Shakir, who is presented as a 'researcher in the sciences of I`jaz in the Qur'an and the Sunna' quotes an obscure hair beautician he refers to as Olga Kokhas as saying 'With the appearance of the corona disease, myths have spread, one of which is that for facial masks to be more effective, all hair should be shaved from the face; however, the coronavirus is so small that it penetrates the skin; thus, beards can protect the skin from the virus, provided the beard is regularly washed and cleaned.' He adds: 'On this the Prophet (Peace Be Upon Him) said: 'cut moustaches and let beards [grow], depart from the polytheists.' It appears that growing beards and cleaning them with water in ablution is an effective prophetic practice.' This kind of statement does not merit a rebuttal, and were it not for its social consumption and impact, it should certainly not be paid any attention to.

Conclusion

The theological questions raised by Covid-19, its meaning and purpose, will continue to be debated. If this is a divine act, for it surely could not be a random event, being of such magnitude, is it a test or a punishment? Is it an act or a message to a particular group or to the whole world? How should one reply to Muslims who are filled with doubts about the value and meaning of faith altogether, finding it difficult to make sense of the crisis (if it is divine in nature) and seeing everyone turning to and seeking help solely from scientists. Islamic scholars also struggled with the response question: what roles should faith, prayer and supplications, but also reason, science and medicine, psychology and sociology, play in the way Muslims and humans should act (or react)? Can religious practices (collective prayers, rituals, etc.) evolve, temporarily or permanently, in response to these unprecedented circumstances, or should tradition still be a reference for religious activities?

And if these questions were not enough on Muslims' plates, additional, idiosyncratic issues were raised in connection to recent Islamic trends: I`jaz and pseudoscience.

Indeed, despite the growing resistance to the phenomenon of I`jaz (the 'miraculous scientific contents in the Qur'an and the Sunna, the Prophetic Tradition'), Covid-19 gave it a new impetus, as some proponents of I`jaz found 'references' to it in the Qur'an or interpreted some hadiths as being prescient – another case of 'Prophetic I`jaz'. Yet, as far back as the fourteenth century, scholars such as the historian and sociologist Ibn Khaldun had explained that the 'Prophetic medicine' was nothing more than 'Bedouin medicine' with no religious connotation or implication whatsoever. In fact, in other cases, social or health-related advice given by the Prophet (for example, camel urine and bloodletting) has been challenged, not validated, by medicine.

Muslim popular discourse has also relied heavily on pseudoscience to promote Islamic rituals (ablution, fasting) or alleged traditions (eating seven dates) as having great value in the prevention or the treatment of Covid-19. Unfortunately, social media greatly helped spread such pseudoscientific claims, illogical thinking, and irrational discourse. The crisis has raised several important and interesting issues, and it will fuel research and discussions, as well as popular misconceptions, for years to come.

SWOLLEN FEET

Chandrika Parmar

India's first case of novel coronavirus was detected on 30 January 2020 in the State of Kerala. As the number of confirmed Covid-19 positive cases started to increase the government clamped Epidemic Diseases Act 1897 on 11 March 2020. Then came the announcement of 'Janta curfew' on 22 March. The Indian railways decided to stop all passenger trains beginning at midnight on 23 March. On the same day India's prime minister, Narendra Modi, in his address to the nation announced a twenty-one-day lockdown to combat the spread of the virus. Except for essential services, all commercial, industrial, religious and cultural activity was to stop. India also shut down the transport services: city and state buses, local transportation, domestic flights, were all suspended. Residents were required to stay home. Most states also sealed their borders restricting movement within and in between states. 'Stay home, stay safe' became the slogan.

The idea of lockdown had already been experimented with in China before it travelled to India. Several other Asian countries from Japan, to South Korea, Vietnam, and Taiwan had recommended and experimented with variants of localised and regional lockdowns to combat the coronavirus. Italy had become the first European country to travel down the route of lockdown. China, the first country to experience a Covid-19 outbreak, had shut down the city of Wuhan, the epicentre of the outbreak, and then closed large parts of the country. Its efforts earned China praise from The World Health Organization as 'perhaps the most ambitious, agile and aggressive disease containment effort in history'. But the lockdown in India was even bigger. Its three-week lockdown would directly affect 1.3 billion people; it would be extended two times more. The first lockdown was between 23 March and 14 April. The second, extended lockdown covered 15 April to 3 May. And the third, from 4 May to 17 May.

The lockdown triggered the second biggest migration in the history of India. There are an estimated 139 million migrants in India – men, women and children, mostly daily wage workers, who leave their homes to seek work and employment far and wide throughout India. Suddenly these migrants were trapped without work, with no money, far away from home. The poignancy of the first migration, due to partition, is obvious. But the poetics of the second has to be seen by foraging through the stories of those who had to travel back to their homes.

The first images of the lockdown to filter through were largely on social media. They were of the policemen with the *lathi*. Anyone violating the 'lockdown' was dealt with 'severely'. There were multiple videos and reports of police assaults and beatings, and, in some cases, even opening fire at people breaking the lockdown rules. On one incident a middle-aged man was shot in the leg by the police. In another incident nineteen-year-old Mohammed Rizwan, resident of Chhajjapur village in Uttar Pradesh went out of his home to buy biscuits. He was beaten up with rifle butts and *lathis* by a group of policemen. He reached home injured. He died in a local hospital on 18 April. In Mumbai a petition was filed by Firdause Irani, raising concerns on police brutality amid the lockdown. Irani's counsel Gopal Sankarnarayan told the court that they had thirteen videos showing police excesses on people while imposing the lockdown orders. 'Policemen are seen assaulting people with *lathis* or slapping them without first asking the reason why they are travelling' he argued. The high court, however, said there are two sides to the story. 'Police brutality is only one side of the coin. The truth is that there are many amongst us who do not care about the lockdown guidelines and do not comply with restrictions. There are black sheep everywhere, Chief Justice Datta added. So who were the black sheep?

Most migrants faced hunger or homelessness if they could not work. The survey by Stranded Workers Action Network (SWAN) of 11,000 migrants found that the average daily wage prior to lockdown was Rs 402 (median daily wage was Rs 400), and about 70 per cent of them were left with less than Rs 200 (less than half their daily wages) for the remaining lockdown period. The survey revealed an intense and urgent hunger crisis. Fifty per cent of the workers had rations left for less than one day. Seventy-two per cent of the people the SWAN team spoke to said that their rations would finish in two days. Because they had little or no cash in hand and were continuously beset by uncertainty about the next meal, many had been eating frugally. A group of 240 workers in Bengaluru told SWAN, 'We are eating only one meal a day to conserve the quantum of grain we have.'

The SWAN report cites several cases where people were already on the brink of starvation. Sujit Kumar, a worker from Bihar stranded in Bhatinda, Punjab, had not eaten in four days. Yasmeen, a tenth standard student in Noida said, 'we have four babies in the house for whom we need milk; we have been feeding them sugar water these days'.

I started getting several distress calls from villagers and acquaintances indicating they had no money and no rations. Abdul, a carer who had once worked with my late uncle, called saying he and four roommates had been stuck in their room for more than one week with no rations. He had reached out in desperation. Rampukar Pandit, a construction labourer, who worked at a cinema hall site in Delhi, was spotted weeping uncontrollably as he talked on the phone by the side of the Nizamuddin Bridge in Delhi. He had broken down at not being able to meet his son before he died. His photograph by PTI photographer Atul Yadav became a snapshot of India's migrant tragedy. 'We labourers have no life, we are just a cog in the wheel, spinning continuously until we run out of life.... My wife, who is unwell, and my three daughters, Poonam (9), Pooja (4) and Priti (2) are waiting for me. The wait just doesn't seem to end,' he told *Indian Express.* Account after account from different social sector organisations document the plight of the labourers, the migrants. Eventually, it is like one giant canvas composed of overlapping miniatures each one provides a vernacular of suffering which merges into the wider normal of forced migration.

I soon realised that highways and side roads connecting cities had become theatre for the tragedy. A walk is now a test of suffering. A walk also becomes a lesson in waiting.

Vinod Yadav, who did plaster work for houses in Bangalore, had not been paid in weeks when he decided to walk. 'We came back crying,' he said. Before lockdown, he would make Rs 300 a day painting houses but as the source of income dried up, he had no choice but to head home on foot to UP.

The Chhattisgarh-based social activist, Priyanka Shukla, documented the travel of about one thousand migrant workers. She describes some of their stories. Sataria Hembrom, thirty-one years old, walked back to his village in Jharkhand's Chaibasa from Mumbai, a distance of more than 1,800 kilometres, with six others. All seven worked at a construction site in Navi Mumbai, where the work stopped on 22 March. Initially, they bought food from their savings, and managed to survive for a month. Then they started running low on money. 'We had two options: face Covid without food or walk home'. They started their journey on 2 May and ended it on 13 May, walking and hitching rides. Shukla says migrants crossing Bilaspur, in the state of Chhattisgarh, is an everyday event. 'About 200 workers cross Bilaspur every night on foot or cycling as they avoid the heat of the day. They are from Jharkhand, Uttar Pradesh, Madhya Pradesh and are coming from the southern states and Maharashtra. Many of the workers have no money; whatever they have, including savings, goes towards food, and to pay truck and bus drivers'.

It was a horrible journey. 'One man fell down from the truck and hurt himself,' recalled Lakshmi Morya, an autorickshaw driver, who paid Rs 3,000 to a truck driver, to travel back to his village in Hardoi district of Uttar Pradesh. He arrived on 13 May, four days after starting from Goregaon in Mumbai, with seventy other people, all packed into the goods compartment of a truck. Joshana S, a resident of Pratiksha Nagar in Mumbai's Sion, said two of her brothers-in-law had already left for Kanpur in trucks and two other relatives were leaving soon. 'It is getting difficult to survive in Mumbai with no income for two months and all work avenues closed,' she said.

Not all were on the road though. Many workers continued to languish in camps. *The Print* covered a story at the Commercial Building of Sadar Bazar where some 400 homeless people and workers doing menial jobs were locked into Night Shelter Number 28. When they were discovered by a reporter on 27 March, he found that men, women and children inside the facility had gathered at the gate and were shaking it. Among the women was a pregnant twenty year-old Chandni, wife of a labourer who earns Rs 300-400 a day. 'Tomorrow, I will complete nine months of my pregnancy. I'm due any day now,' she said from behind the locked gate, holding her swollen belly. 'Do they expect me to give birth here? We have been caged without food'. Chandni, like everyone else in the facility, had not seen a doctor since the lockdown was announced. She would normally go to a free clinic at Lady Hardinge hospital in Connaught Place for regular consultations but was not able to follow up for the past five days. 'Our income has stopped and no one has come to feed us, either. I haven't eaten properly. How am I going to give birth?' Chandni wondered. The families in this facility – including at least three pregnant women – had gone without food for three days before a ration of *atta* and *dal* was delivered to them. No one had explained to the families exactly what the coronavirus is. 'Beyond the name, we don't know what it is,' said sixty-year-old Saholi

Hunger and starvation became one of the most haunting pictures on social media. The mainstream media carried images of men and women walking with their belongings on their heads and shoulders. Of mothers walking carrying a sleeping baby on their shoulders. Sometimes it was an image of the man pushing his pregnant wife and child and their belongings in a rented cart. Or children wailing in pain as their feet hurt while they were dragged along by their parents. Rani Punnaserril, a member of the Sisters of the Holy Cross, spoke of Rajesh, a migrant, who had reached out to ask her for food. He was so emotional that he could not even speak. He said, 'my children are crying for food. I have nothing to give them. Police are chasing us away if we go to the road to collect something to eat'. But pictures give a two dimensional understanding of starvation. One has to realise that the migrants are literally confined to spaces. Rather than becoming a refuge, in many cases, these spaces virtually stifled both liberty and agency.

The stories of pain and suffering repeat themselves as if to echo the very repetitiveness of walking. The tiredness of the swollen feet echo in the very tiredness and abruptness of narratives.

Sudarshan Saharkar in his article on PARI (Peoples Archive for Rural India) tells similar stories. He lists how a large number of migrants had to pass through Nagpur in the centre of the country. As he puts it, 'they came every day, on foot, on bicycles, on trucks, in buses, in or on just about any vehicles they could find. Tired, exhausted, desperate to reach home. Men and women of all ages, many children, too.' He goes on to list those passing through. A young couple with their forty-four-day-old baby girl, travelling from Hyderabad to Gorakhpur, on a hired motorbike, in temperatures touching the mid-forties. Thirty-four young women from villages in Chhattisgarh's Dhamtari district, trying to reach home from Ahmedabad where they had gone to train under a skill development programme.

Five young men, on their recently purchased bicycles, heading for Rayagada district of Odisha. On the outer ring road of Nagpur, hundreds of migrants arrive from National Highways 6 and 7, each day. They are served food at several points and find shelters around a toll plaza, organised by the district administration and a coalition of NGOs and citizens' groups. The labourers rest through the scorching summer day and resume their journeys by evening. Journalist Ispita Chakravarty writes in her Scroll.in article, 'across the country, there are men and women with swollen feet'. She talks of seventeen-year-old Baliram Kumar at a quarantine centre in Uttar Pradesh's Gorakhpur district, who had walked from Bangalore for over twenty-five days. His feet were cut and scabbed. His whole body ached. At another quarantine centre in the village school, in Bihar's Katihar district, there is twenty-year-old Vinod Yadav. By the time he reached his village, in the late-May heat, it had been twenty-seven days since he left Bangalore. The list and images are endless. The suffering of the body politic is virtually caught in the pain of the feet. Swollen feet become a metaphor for the overall tales of suffering. A blister in that sense becomes an everyday memorial to the anonymity of pain.

Joyti Kumari, at the tender age of fifteen, cycled 745 kilometres from Gurgaon, Haryana, to Darbhanga, Bihar with her injured father on the cycle carrier. Jyoti's father, Mohan Paswan, had been an auto rickshaw driver in Gurgaon for twenty years. He met with an accident. Jyoti with her mother came to Gurgaon to take care of him. As Jyoti's mother, Phoolo Devi, was working in an Anganwadi as a cook, she could not stay in Gurgaon for long. She returned to Darbhanga, leaving Jyoti behind to look after her father. Lockdown happened. Her father had no source of income and they were running out of rations. Soon, they were left with no money to pay rent. 'Problems increased after the lockdown,' says Jyoti. 'Our landlord wanted to throw us out of the rented room. He had even cut the power twice as we hadn't paid the rent. We had also run out of rations. What would we have eaten? Father had no income at all, so we thought of returning home somehow.' Jyoti persuaded her father to buy a bicycle with the remaining money. On 8 May, she started from Gurgaon with her father on the bicycle's carrier for her long and painful trek.

Another episode that garnered considerable attention was the story of two friends, Mohammed Saiyub, twenty-three, and Amrit Kumar, twenty-four. They were part of a group that was heading to Uttar Pradesh from Surat, Gujarat. According to reports they were friends since childhood, the two had left the village hoping to earn a better living in the city – Saiyub was the first to leave, for Mumbai, while Amrit went to Surat. Around three years ago, Amrit convinced Saiyub to shift to Surat too. They worked in different textile units but shared a room. They both boarded a truck to travel back to their village. On the way Amrit felt nauseous. A fellow passenger suspecting the worst asked him to get out of the truck. Concerned about how his ailing friend would manage, Saiyub also alighted, at Shivpuri. Keeping Amrit's head in his lap, he walked crying along the Shivpuri highway seeking help. Their photograph would take social media by storm. Amrit had to be put on a ventilator but he passed away. He tested negative for Covid-19. Shivpuri Chief Medical and Health Officer Dr AL Sharma said Amrit's lungs were clear but he had severe dehydration.

The pain and suffering seen everywhere was invisible to the state. On 31 March, the Supreme Court heard a petition filed by lawyer AA Srivastava seeking directions to provide food and shelter to migrant workers amid the coronavirus lockdown. Solicitor General Tushar Mehta in his response told the Supreme Court that there was a complete prohibition on interstate migration, and around 23,000 had been provided with food, which included migrants and daily wagers. The central government told the Supreme Court 'no one is on the road. They [migrant workers] have been taken to the nearest available shelter'.

The news channels, however, continued to report and show live streams of migrants on the road. Even as late as the third week of May, there were reports of 'migrants' sleeping on the pavement. Thousands of them who had been employed in non-construction sectors like hotels, malls, or even as street vendors – all of which had been closed by then. With no money to pay rent, they had been evicted by landlords. An increasing number had taken to sleeping on pavements or in makeshift camps driven by the lack of jobs, hunger and homelessness. Satyam Kumar, a mason from Bihar who was residing in Sudhamanagar in Karnataka says: 'the landlord evicted twenty of us from a room for non-payment of rent. He had given us a deadline of 5 May. After that, he cut water and power supply'. Karim Laskar, a carpenter from West Bengal, tells a similar story: 'we mostly stay on site and move to a new project once work is completed. Our engagement with projects is for a short duration. While we continued to work during the lockdown on the project we were engaged in, once our work was completed, we had to move out of that site. But we are not getting new projects, which has rendered us homeless'. A group of forty-eight migrant labourers, evicted by their landlords, including one in an advanced stage of pregnancy, were forced to set out on a 1,000-kilometre trek home to Madhya Pradesh from Haryana's Ambala. In another widely reported story, twenty-eight-year-old Maan Kumari gave birth on the roadside somewhere between Ambala and Aligarh and then walked at least 150 kilometres, braving the summer sun and thunderstorms, with her new-born in her arms. In yet another story covered extensively by the media a young migrant worker from Madhya Pradesh started his tough journey from Hyderabad along with his pregnant wife, Dhanwanta, and infant daughter, Anuragini. He wheeled his daughter and pregnant wife for the most part of the 700-kilometre route on a makeshift wooden cart that he made with wood and sticks. A desperate migrant worker stole a bicycle in Rajasthan's Bharatpur to pedal his way to home in Uttar Pradesh, covering a distance of more than 250 kilometres. The man left behind an apology note, explaining his situation: '*Main majdoor hun, majboor bhi. Main aapka gunehgar hu. Aapki cycle lekar ja raha hu. Mujhe maaf kar dena. Mujhe Bareily tak jana he. Mere pass koi sadhan nahi he aur viklang baccha hai*,' read the note written in Hindi. 'I'm a labourer and also helpless. I'm your culprit too. I'm taking your bicycle. Please forgive me. I have no other means to reach my home, and I have a disabled child. I have to go to Bareilly'.

The migrants have few storytellers. Only a few journalists followed their predicament with persistence and commitment. One of those who did is Barkha Dutt, a television reporter, columnist on *The Hindustan Times* and owner of the YouTube news channel MoJo. Dutt systematically pursued the plight of the migrant, following the workers in the blistering heat of April and May. In a candid interview she admits that she stepped out with a sense of curiosity to see what was happening. What she saw and experienced changed her from being an advocate of the lockdown to a strong opponent. In one of the early encounters she came across a family of six. They were walking 'home' in the scorching heat. She caught up with them as Seema and Prem stopped to drink water from a pipe where water was leaking. They were walking to Mohammadpur in Uttar Pradesh from Haryana. Two children of ten and twelve walked while two younger ones aged five and four were carried by their parents. Their only refrain was 'we want to reach our house but when I reach back home, I don't know how I will feed my children'. It was poignant to watch the two children holding onto their blistered feet and telling the reporter: '*hum chalte chalte thak gaye hain*' (We are tired, just walking, and walking). She spoke to the young child Pallavi who told her 'My dream is that I will never be poor' Another child she spoke to told her that coronavirus '*matlab hai ki humme khana nahi milega*' (means we will not get food). She found eighty-year-old Leelavati abandoned on Bandra station in Mumbai by her son. Many migrants told her 'poverty will kill us before the virus'. A common plea was '*kahi pe kaam miljayega*' – where can we get some work.

Several images will stay with me for years whenever I think of the lockdown-induced migrant crisis. The haunting image, for example, of the mowing down of sixteen migrants sleeping on a railway track in Aurangabad, Maharashtra. Railway tracks, often as part of folklore, are perceived to be the shortest route to the destination. Throughout the lockdown, migrants walked along railway tracks to avoid highways or police brutality on the roads. The incident took place on 7 May. The migrants, who had walked 36 kilometres on the first stretch of what would have been their journey home to Madhya Pradesh, had fallen asleep on the railway track. A goods train ploughed through them at daybreak. A heart-wrenching video surfaced on social media on 25 May which shows a child trying to wake his dead mother at a railway platform in Bihar's Muzaffarpur. He can also be seen tugging at the blanket and then covering his own head with it as his mother lay still. The thirty-five-year-old migrant woman, Avreena Khatoon, reportedly died of hunger and dehydration while travelling to Muzaffarpur from Ahmedabad in a Shramik Special train. Jamalo Madkam, a twelve-year-old Adivasi girl was walking home to Chattisgarh from the chilli fields of Telangana. She walked 140 kilometres in three days and finally collapsed and died due to exhaustion, dehydration and muscle fatigue, 60 kilometres away from her home. She had gone to the chilli fields as a labourer. With lockdown the work stopped. With no transport she along with the other labourers started walking back to the village 200 kilometres away. She died on 18 April. In Delhi, outside Night Shelter Number 101, at Yamuna Pushta near the Nigambodh Ghat cremation ground, a man lay on the pavement of a deserted street, scarcely moving. Flies collected near his face as a crowd of migrant labourers watched. 'Can you tell us if he is alive or dead?', someone asked. 'This is what happens when you let us starve. He had been ill for many days and has not eaten,' said one of the labourers who wanted a place at the shelter.

For almost a month, the only way the workers could return home was by walking, cycling, or hitching rides. Then, a few state governments started organising buses. In late April, the central government came out with a protocol on inter-state movement of migrants on buses – all inter-state movement had been barred until then, and then, perhaps realising that trains were faster, safer, and could accommodate more, finally started running special Shramik trains on 1 May, International Workers' Day.

What happened when the migrant workers returned home? The agony of walking was over. The evicted workers then found themselves homeless at home. No longer the suppliers of remittances but instead, individuals marked by stigma as virus 'carriers'. Quarantine camps become substitutes for homes. Many labourers returned home to Bihar and UP only to find that they were not welcome. Many of the social sector partners I spoke to described the stigma being faced by the 'migrants' returning home from the city. So much was the fear and shame associated with coronavirus that in many cases the returning migrants were reported and the villagers handed them over to the police, who put them into quarantine camps. In some bizarre cases, returning villagers in Bareilly, Uttar Pradesh were sprayed with chemicals to disinfectant them.

The Covid crisis has shown that migrant workers only retain a liminal form of citizenship. They are creatures unwelcome at their original home and treated ambiguously at the point of destination. The very spraying of migrants with chemicals projected them as vermin, subject to harassment by police officers, clerks, landlords, factories, railway officials, state bureaucrats, courts and the government. Many, many died during their homeward journeys: burned to death in forest fires, being hit or crushed by truck/bus/trains, exhaustion, heart attack, vomiting blood, chest pain, asphyxiation after falling in a deep pit, being trapped in snow, stomach pain, breathlessness, hunger, exhaustion, dehydration, fatigue, multi-organ failure, and snake bites. But who cares about the deaths of rodents?

On 14 September 2020, the Narendra Modi government informed Parliament that it had not maintained any data on the number of migrant workers who died while trying to reach their homes after the nationwide lockdown was announced. Lok Sabha MPs K Navaskani, Suresh Narayan Dhanorkar, and Adoor Prakash, had asked the Modi government if it was aware that a number of migrant workers had lost their lives during their return to their hometowns. The MPs also sought to know if the government had provided any compensation or economic assistance to the victims' families. To this, the Union Ministry for Labour and Employment gave a written reply: 'no such data is maintained'; and the answer to the question on compensation 'does not arise' since there is no data.

The suffering and pain is not just the litany of endless walking. It is the indifference and callousness with which the workers were treated. Some of these narratives of evicted labourers capture the poetics and poignancy of the 1943 Bengal famine. But the hunger and desperation of the lockdown was so visible yet so invisible. The density and the intensity of what actually happens cannot be caught in announcement of lockdowns. Lockdowns substitute the idea of law and order for governance. Governance caters to citizenship. It is this indifference that becomes obvious in the stories of those who suffer.

IRANIAN DILEMMAS

Lila Randall

Iranian scientists are in a political quagmire. Eight months of deceitful coronavirus guidance has shattered the regime's authority. A new virus has swept across Iran: distrust.

Covid-19 has struck during a very crucial era in Iran. In 2019, public confidence in Iranian authorities was crushed when demonstrations over petrol prices in more than one hundred cities resulted in over 1,500 deaths, and the Iranian Revolutionary Guards Corps used missiles to shoot down a Ukraine International Airlines Flight 752 in Tehran. When the coronavirus first swept across the nation in February 2020, the government prioritised political aims. A calendar of events made social distancing – the most effective means of controlling the virus – all the more difficult. These included the celebrations marking the parliamentary elections on 21 February, the revolution's anniversary on 11 February and Nowruz – the Iranian New Year on 20 March.

Officials first reported the deaths of Iranians on 19 February – but reports say cases entered the country at least ten days earlier by passengers travelling on Mahan Airlines from Wuhan, where the outbreak began. The government opposed full national lockdowns citing economic constraints in rural and lower income urban areas as another reason to avoid a ban on movement. Religious authorities in the holy city of Qom, located some 130 kilometres from the capital city of Tehran, refused to close holy shrines. They believed sacred protection would prevent the virus spreading. The Iranian administration failed to identify and isolate people who came into contact with the virus. Officials could not convince the clergy in Qom the situation was grave enough to take immediate social distancing measures to stop transmission of the virus.

Without trust, a society cannot function smoothly. Social scientists have linked the declining trust in healthcare – and the media – with broader epistemological challenges about the authenticity of knowledge, confidence in the power of science, and the capacity of medics to deliver control over our bodies. As political economist Robert Crawford notes, 'when the life-world is colonised by medical insecurity, medicalised subjects come to suspect the messenger and the knowledge they bear'; leading to a breakdown in communication between the medical profession and citizens. Now Iranians are freestyling; they flout the rules by keeping businesses open, host gatherings, and travel 'more than ever'.

Mojtaba Pourmohsen, a journalist at Iran International TV, who was sentenced to one-year in prison in 2009 for alleged propaganda against the regime, said citizens don't know what advice is sound. Speaking over the phone, he told me: 'citizens feel they cannot rely on the Government, the regime, nor the health and medical advice they receive from international organisations working in the country'.

Few events thrust into view the hardiness of a healthcare system than an international outbreak of a deadly virus. Since the 1979 Islamic revolution, Iran has been largely successful in improving the overall health of citizens in rural and urban areas. Yet the system suffers crippling flaws that make it ill-prepared to deal with a pandemic of this scale. The overall nature of the healthcare system focuses on primary care – but a pandemic such as this demands the more advanced secondary and tertiary. The latter requires more cutting-edge medical equipment and treatment.

Most notably, by focusing on primary healthcare, services have become outdated and have neglected changes in the patterns of diseases. Emphasis remains on providing treatment for illness rather than advocating preventative health and hygiene, as can be seen in Iran's struggle with the virus today. Citizens have reported problems buying masks and sanitisers, both because of shortage and the price of goods jumping tenfold.

The changing needs of Iranian society is not reflected in the care available. The increase in the number of hospital beds does not mirror the growth in population. Since the Islamic Republic first established a health network in 1984, later expanded in 2005, rural-urban migration has rocketed and densely populated areas on the outskirts of cities were strained with a limit in hospital beds even before the pandemic. Hospitals have reportedly been short on equipment like testing kits throughout.

'For a while there was rumours that people were dying and that nobody knows why. Doctors were seeing patients with atypical pneumonia and very severe cases but they had no clue what it was and there was no test available', said Shahram Kordrastri, a haematologist and lecturer at King's College London, who works closely with scientists in Iran.

China and European nations donated medical equipment under humanitarian mechanisms to Iran to bypass the US sanctions. Popular rumours on the whereabouts of these supplies claim – and these have not been verified – that the Islamic Revolutionary Guard Corps (IRGC) redirected supplies like diagnostic kits, ventilators, PPE, such as gloves and masks, to their own hospitals for officials to use leaving the public facilities scantily equipped. A shortage of drugs and medical equipment exacerbates other issues. Like most big bureaucracies, Iran's healthcare system has a history of nepotism and corruption. One source, an exiled journalist, said: 'Iran uses coronavirus aid to treat members of the regime at IRGC hospitals. Citizens aren't seeing any progress in the support offered to people in hospital'. And a medical professional in Tehran adds: 'scarcity has opened the door to hoarding and profiteering, often with the collusion of officials and regulators who are hard pressed like everyone else. We are witnessing the delegitimisation of the entire system as ordinary people face medicine shortages and exorbitant prices'.

In July 2020, Iran's Minister of Health, Saeed Namaki, warned of possible uprisings from the lower classes due to the economic pressure of coronavirus and called for security forces to introduce preventative measures. Although the healthcare system was evolved in 2005 to decrease inequalities in the quality of care, economic division has tainted citizens' experience during the pandemic. In wealthier cities such as Tehran, supermarkets hand out PPE like free gloves and sanitisers to customers upon entry. No food shortages have been reported and medical facilities are accessible with no queues. The behaviour and expectations of the health-aware and well-informed middle classes remains worlds apart from the majority. 'It's a black-market. If you have enough money you can easily find the testing kits and hospital equipment. High-end shops and supermarkets also have higher cleanliness standards in response to the virus', Kordrastri added.

Pourmohsen said in many areas people have grown tired of the economic burden of the virus, including in Gilan, where he worked as an editor-in-chief at *Gilan-e Emrouz* before he angered authorities with an interview with an 'anti-revolutionary' gay poet. With more than 13.3 million in Iran living below the poverty line – getting the right service is a gamble for many.

'The Metro and buses (in Gilan) were full of people, mostly without masks. The government has not had a support program for covering business or families that have been harmed by Covid-19. The price of drugs has been very high. People have to buy them from black market at more than fifty times higher price', Pourmohsen added. Hospitals in Gilan were overcrowded and lacked medical equipment earlier this year, according to Pourmohsen, who once lived in Rasht, the capital city of Gilan Province, which, at the time of writing, is in the high-risk 'red zone' having consistently had a high number of cases.

As Covid-19 hit, scientists joined the global race to develop a vaccine fearing US sanctions would impede their ability to import one. The sanctions, brought in during 2018, impact all trade and transactions with Iran and have had a devastating effect on healthcare. From causing problems in importing some of the ingredients needed for domestically producing drugs to securing financial support from international banks, insurance firms and getting financial institutions to underwrite medical imports – the sanctions drastically hamper Iranians. Pharmaceutical and medical supplies are technically exempt from the sanction's regime, but suppliers are often reluctant to work with Iranian vendors over concerns of crossing the terms of the US sanctions. Drugs already inside the country are often sold at inflated prices, and can be of an inferior quality. Within a month of the outbreak, some medical professionals campaigned to the UN Secretary General Antonio Guterres for the removal of the sanctions. They claimed the sanctions had directly contributed towards the death of eighty healthcare workers.

For the vaccine, researchers launched forty-five clinical trials in a bid to find a suitable treatment. Communicating via email, Dr Reza Malekzadeh, deputy minister of health and medical education for research and technology, and Director at the Digestive Disease Research Institute at Tehran University, said interim results show the most effective drugs in their trials are Remdesvir, first developed to fight Ebola, and the hepatitis C treatment, Sofosbuvr. Tehran Univeristy of Medical Sciences is overseeing the testing of Remdesvir with thirty hospitals across the country carrying out a randomised trial. The drug has produced conflicting reports after it flopped in its first trial. But the medication, developed by Gilead Sciences of Foster City, California, has bounced back after trials showed it could shorten the recovery time of Covid patients. Malekzadeh said scientists are not only searching for a treatment for Covid-19 but are also putting down foundations for future outbreaks. 'We are trying our best to find the most effective and safe treatment for coronavirus. We are very hopeful that we, along with other scientists across the globe, will find effective therapy and vaccine for this Covid-19 infection and become ready for future similar epidemics', he said.

Sofosbuvir, or Sovaldi, is the country's second most promising drug. Eight clinical trials were carried out during 2020 to test various combinations of it, with enthusiasm for the drug rooted in its ability to prevent the replication of infected cells. Malekzadeh added that scientists are monitoring a new strain of coronavirus to see if it will become dominant around the world. The mutated form of SARS-CoV-2, known as a 382-nucleotide deletion, displays weaker, less threatening, symptoms than the current dominant strain known as 'wild'. If the mutated virus takes over, more people would experience milder symptoms such as a lower temperature and fewer patients would need oxygen support. He added: 'we don't know yet if this strain will overtake'. If it does, it could mean a huge drop in hospitalisations. Other notable differences in those who had the mutation are that the infected are younger overall. In the study of 432 individuals diagnosed in Singapore with coronavirus between 22 January and 21 March 2020, only three per cent of the participants were aged sixty-five or older.

Patients in countries including Singapore, Bangladesh, Australia and Spain were found to have the mutated virus as early as January and February when it was first announced the coronavirus had spread globally. The study was published in August 2020 and carried out by a large group of Singaporean institutes, hospitals and laboratories including the Department of Infectious Diseases and National Public Health Laboratory. In October, hospitals in Iran announced they would not treat nonemergency patients as they were unable to cope with the high number of admissions. Military hospitals also opened their doors to admit civilian coronavirus patients. Other countries had already taken similar measures last year but it was the first time for Iran.

A doctor working in Kashan, a city in the province of Isfahan, who doesn't want to be identified, told me, via WhatsApp, that the healthcare network set up for Covid in his region had been successful. From February to March, he said they hadn't witnessed a shortage of staff but medics had grown tired and were anxious about the number of beds available in the coming months. The mutated virus could improve patient's overall recovery – freeing up hospital beds. By December 2020, two per cent of the population – 5,809 people – were in a serious or critical condition requiring intensive care.

Injury to the lungs shocked the medical profession in Iran. One doctor described the scarring and structural damage to the lungs, as looking like a 'bomb blast has gone off'. Another doctor, who referred to himself only as Azad, carried out a CT scan and chest X-rays on a Covid patient, who succumbed to the virus before a treatment plan could be decided. 'I'd never seen anything like it before,' Azad said, noting the severity of the injury.

Iranians have a long history of favouring alternative medicines for treating ailments. The full list of clinical trials spans all kinds of medicine, including traditional pharmaceutical and natural, herbal, combinations. One clinical trial is testing the homeopathic remedy, ipecac, prescribed for dry, irritated coughs, wheezy breathing and stubborn phlegm – all common symptoms of the coronavirus. Another is a herbal drink of marshmallow and liquorice. Marshmallow is praised for reducing swelling in the mucous membranes that line the respiratory tract and Liquorice is hailed for its immune boosting properties. Presumably this one was put to the test after recovery from the coronavirus was found to be largely dependent on the patient's immune response.

Once a vaccine becomes available in Iran, the next battle could be encouraging citizens to take it. After news of a vaccine in other countries, such as the UK, popular support for the vaccine dwindled just at it began being rolled out in December. A third of Britons said they are either unsure or definitely wouldn't use a vaccine for coronavirus. But online anti-vaccine misinformation is unlikely to enter Iran which has a long history of censorship particularly at times of unrest. Iranians have grown used to internet restrictions with tens of thousands of websites censored, according to a 2017 report from the watchdog Freedom House. That includes the websites of foreign news outlets, human rights organisations, political opposition groups and others not aligned with the theocratic regime. Popular social networks such as Facebook, Twitter and YouTube and the blogging platforms WordPress and Blogger are also monitored. This wasn't always the way.

In the remaining weeks of the Shah's rule before the Islamic revolution in 1979, Iranians witnessed a period of relative freedom. Media outlets reported freely just as an air of independence and choice coloured the daily lives of Iranians. It was at this time, the country signed up to the first of the United Nations international human rights treaties, binding it to facilitate freedom of expression, the free flow of information and pluralism of the media (Article 19 of the ICCPR and the Universal Declaration of Human Rights both protect freedom of expression). These contracts have been broken countless times since – and authorities are pushing for stricter censorship.

In August 2019, a consortium of forty lawmakers in Iran proposed a controversial draft bill to the parliament that could result in harsher online censorship. It would see the armed forces, including the IRGC controlling Internet gateways. The Bill has also called for the creation of a board to oversee social media platforms and to manage violations of internet use such as the spreading of coronavirus disinformation. The board would be made up of representatives from government, the judiciary and the IRGC's feared Intelligence Unit which has arrested scores of journalists, activists and environmentalists in recent years.

Aggressive censorship makes sourcing valuable information from the country somewhat difficult. After eight months of contact-building, emails, WhatsApp messages and phone calls – the total number frustratingly high – communications with scientists, academics and politicians remain *redacted.* From the end of March 2020, the regime monitored the mobile phones of scientists, while Iran's Coronavirus Combat Taskforce suspended all newspaper printing delivery and distribution in April citing the need to stop the virus being transmitted via the inks. My contacts turned silent overnight.

Dealing with a pandemic is no small feat for any government. But the challenges Iran's scientists now face begs the question, how do you dissolve tension between citizens and authority when trust has been obliterated. Should governments conceal some information to prevent pandemonium? For some, gaining public trust means engaging citizens in a decision-making process that is transparent, pluralistic and participatory. An unlikely prospect for Iran. One thing seems sure: the country will not overcome its battle with Covid-19 if trust in the medical profession is not restored.

VIRAL DREAMS

Leyla Jagiella

'A lion cannot hunt his game,
If he does not leave his forest, his narrow plain.
If an arrow does not leave the bow,
It will never reach its aim.'

This poem is one of many ascribed to 'Ali ibn Abi Talib, the relative and son-in-law of the Prophet Muhammad, respected as the fourth Rightly Guided Caliph by all Sunni Muslims, revered as the first divinely appointed Imam by Shi'a Muslims, and viewed as a fountain of spiritual knowledge and the primary transmitter of the mystical teachings of the Prophet by many Sufis. In the so-called *Diwan of `Ali ibn Abi Talib*, these poetic lines are given the title of 'On the Benefits of Travelling', stressing the importance that journeying and travelling should have for every human being and most certainly for every Muslim.

If we are not able to travel, than we are like an arrow which has never left its bow. That is indeed a sentiment that I personally relate to very much. And it seems to haunt me in my dreams these days, in these times of a global pandemic that has restricted our ability to travel so much. At least once a week I dream of some impossible trip or journey. Sometimes I dream about a journey taken by train, but much more often I dream of long haul flights. Certainly, I have had dreams like this before as well, once in a while. But never with the same frequency that they seem to occur during my nights of this pandemic period. My subconscious seems to have a very clear idea of what I am missing the most in these times. Not contact with other human beings, not the possibility of heading to the supermarket without having to wear a face-mask, but simply travelling.

There is a part of me that feels a bit disconcerted by these recurring nightly visions. I fear that they might expose my subconscious as one of a far too privileged individual, deeply mourning the loss of an eventually quite elitist exercise that a lot of people on our planet are barred from anyway, pandemic or not. But another part of me tries to reassure myself that this merely shows what a good Muslim subconscious I actually have. Does not our subconscious hold fast to the importance of travelling for every Muslim that Imam Ali has indicated in his poem?

In fact, the importance of travel has not only been stressed by `Ali ibn Abi Talib but has been evoked in Islamic teachings again and again, in many forms. In the Qur'an, God tells us, 'We will show them Our signs in the horizons and in themselves, till it is clear to them that this is the truth' (41:53) and we are taught: 'We created you male and female, and We made you into various nations and tribes, so that you may know each other' (49:13). The Prophet Muhammad is reported to have said: 'Search for knowledge, even if you have to travel as far as China for it.' And, of course, it is worth pointing out that Islam is probably the only global religion that has explicitly made travelling one of its fundamental pillars of religious practice, in the form of the hajj, the pilgrimage to Makkah. Being able to embark on this pilgrimage has always been somewhat of a privilege, of course, and being able to travel has become even more of a privilege these days. But nevertheless, countless Muslims on low-incomes and from deprived backgrounds have dared to, and continue to, undertake this journey.

Beyond the hajj, classical Islam has always celebrated the scholarly ideal of the *rihla `ilmiyya*, the journey in search of knowledge. The precedent for this journey was set by the Prophet Muhammad himself who in his youth accompanied caravans travelling all across the Arab desert from Yemen to Syria. In the classical period, the *rihla `ilmiyya* was put into practice by almost every major intellectual figure of Muslim history; in fact, one was not really taken seriously as a Muslim scholar if one had not left home in search of knowledge at least once.

A Muslim is essentially a traveller, I believe that very strongly. Even those of us who are barred from going on a physical journey due to lack of resources, or due to the circumstances of our lives, or due to the cruelty of passport, borders and visa regimes, are essentially travellers. Our scriptures advise us to always view life as a constant journey and to consider ourselves people who voyage through this world but never truly settle down in it. In our religious practices, we often perform what one could call imaginal journeys: when we pray, we turn towards a distant place in modern day Saudi Arabia, we direct ourselves towards a faraway destination (unless we ourselves live in Saudi Arabia). Traditional Sunni Muslims regularly recite blessings for the Prophet with the understanding that angel wings carry these blessings across borders and nations directly to the illuminated resting place of the Prophet. Shi'a Muslims additionally also often recite *ziyârâts* (literally: visits) to their Imams; they can sit comfortably in their home in London, Dearborn or Skardu and nevertheless 'visit' Imam Husayn in Karbala in Iraq once a week.

Most of us also lead transnational and cosmopolitan everyday lives, constantly in touch with relatives, in-laws and friends all across the globe. It was already a specific hallmark of the Muslim experience in the West for many decades but now, in the days of the pandemic, it has become an even more tangible reality with social media, messenger services and video calls.

We Muslims, therefore, may be seen as a population particularly affected by a world whose borders are becoming increasingly impenetrable and in which both migrating and travelling is becoming more and more arduous. Under the pretence of migration politics, we have already seen a worrying tendency towards increasing restrictions on global movement in recent decades. And the Covid-19 pandemic has now made travelling and migration difficult to an extent that none of us has ever experienced during our lifetimes, certainly not those of us with privileged citizenships and with what has been labelled a 'powerful passport'.

Of course, unlike the madness that has defined Western migration politics in recent years, the reasons for these new Covid-19 restrictions are to a large extent sane and logical, and I even dare say that in many cases these restrictions may not have been enforced enough. I am not complaining about these restrictions on travelling at all. I am sure I can survive without my usual journeys for a year or two. Since I hold on to the imaginal journeys of my faith on the one hand, and to the virtual journeys offered by social media and messenger services on the other. But I still nevertheless miss travelling and that shows in my dreams.

Interestingly, I am not the only person whose dreams have been affected by the pandemic. An astonishing number of people throughout the world have developed a nightly habit of very specific recurring 'pandemic dreams'. According to an article by Tore Nielsen in *Scientific American*, a recent study by a team at Harvard University has found out that 37 per cent of the Americans surveyed had such recurring 'pandemic dreams'. Usually, these dreams were described as nightmares and as rather unsettling, marked by themes of completing impossible tasks and being threatened by others. A large number of people also seem to have developed recurring dreams featuring insects, spiders and other creatures perceived as unclean or dangerous. These creatures may be interpreted as metaphors for the viral threat that we are all exposed to.

I personally have never had any such catastrophic and threatening pandemic dreams. Maybe because, in general, I am coping mentally quite well with the pandemic and all its social and political effects. My subconscious therefore probably does not have any specific axe to grind with me in this situation. I generally sleep well and deeply and am not plagued by nightmares. But there is that strange incidence of repeated dreams about travelling since the pandemic has started and even more so since lockdowns have been enforced on us.

A typical such dream of mine would always involve a long plane journey. I would get terribly excited about the possibility of taking such a long flight. As has also often been the case in my real life, the opportunity to take such a flight often comes connected to an invitation to some conference or arts event abroad. In my dreams, those occasions always show up as a surprise. I didn't actually expect to travel at that time, nor do I personally have the means to do so, but suddenly this opportunity shows up out of the blue. Very often the conference or event takes place in Pakistan, India or Malaysia, countries that I had indeed been travelling to frequently before the pandemic and with which I am connected on many levels. I arrive at the airport. There are no restrictions there, nobody wears a mask, nobody asks me for a Covid-19 test. When the dream runs really well then I also get an upgrade to business class. Something that, in real life, happened once to me and that I have been yearning for ever since. Eventually I sit in the aeroplane and my flight takes off. And then, suddenly, it hits me: I am not supposed to be here! I am not supposed to travel! We are in the middle of a global pandemic and I actually live in a country in lockdown! How did I get here? How did I get to the airport? How did I get on this flight? And that even without wearing a face-mask? And then I usually wake up … and start bemoaning the fact that I am not actually on a business class flight to Asia.

I have had this kind of dream so many times during the last few months that it actually surprises me that each time anew my astral self falls for the deceptive allure of an invitation to a far-away destination and does not seem to remember that this storyline hasn't worked out well a couple of times already. I am usually quite good at remembering other dreams while I am dreaming. My subconscious has even built entire cities that I visit in my dreams again and again and each time I visit these cities I remember my previous visits. There are also three mosques that I visit regularly in my dreams and each time I visit them I notice little changes there and remember that things looked a bit different on my last visit. It sometimes almost seems as if I have an entire parallel life in the imaginal world. Strangely, the airport that I depart from during my 'pandemic dreams' also seems to be a part of that elaborate imaginal world. It is also one of these locations that I return to again and again. It does not look like any airport that I know in real life but nevertheless it has a very distinctive character and appearance that I recognise each time. Being at that airport, I therefore should actually remember my previous failed journeys. But I don`t. Again and again I fall for the promise of a journey and again and again it is only after take-off that I realise that I actually should not be on that flight.

One could describe the dream as a little bit distressing in that I realise that I am in the wrong place at the wrong time. But all in all my pandemic dreams are usually very cheerful. I enjoy being at the airport, I relish the process of boarding, and I just love sitting on an aeroplane seat again and looking forward to reaching an equally familiar and exciting destination soon. This is how I have always felt about flying in real life too. I have always loved air travel. Despite it involving some aspects that do bother me, such as security checks, I have never felt worried or anxious during flights in my whole life and in many ways aeroplanes are a comfort zone for me. And despite my constant yearning for another business class upgrade, I can say that even about the most dubious and challenging flights that I have taken in my life. Even if there are aspects of a journey that others may perceive as worrying and threatening, I often translate these into parts of an exciting adventure for me. Maybe this is just an attitude that I generally have about life. Maybe it is one reason why I am not much negatively affected on a mental level by this pandemic. I treat life in general as an adventurous journey.

I remember very well the first flight that I took. I must have been maybe seven or eight years old, I think, and my parents, my brother and I were flying from Germany to Tunisia. I was very excited to see the world from above for the very first time. The sight of the Mediterranean Sea meeting a coast of date palms is still strongly etched on my mind. I also remember that during this first flight there was some weather turbulence. I asked my mum what this was, why our plane was shaking and jumping so much. She just said, 'Oh, these are just airholes. Doesn't it feel funny how the stomach tickles each time the plane jumps over one of these. Like on a rollercoaster ride at the town fair.' This was probably the best thing one could say to a child in such a situation. And I probably owe it partly to these words that I always associate flying with both comfort and positive excitement.

In fact, I even associate weather turbulences with comfort. I have this very strange habit that everybody else finds quite astonishing: I love turbulence while flying. Not only do I love them, I also sleep exceptionally well while they occur. In fact, I never sleep as well during flights as during those rare occasions when I get a chance to fall asleep during turbulences. People usually call me crazy when I tell them about this idiosyncrasy of mine.

But I think I have found a psychological explanation for this phenomenon that does make some sense. Falling asleep in an aeroplane that is shaking and vibrating probably subconsciously reminds me of being a baby or toddler who is rocked to sleep. It does evoke exactly the kind of warm feeling in me that one can associate with such a memory. In fact, this sensation is so strong in me that often, before departure, I have caught myself thinking 'Oh, I hope there will be turbulences so that I can sleep comfortably'.

Do I not worry for my safety? Am I not concerned for my own life? I have seen faces of people sitting next to me on flights turn green during very soft and tender little jumps that I found perfectly enjoyable. I feel sorry for them. But I feel very different from them. On the rare occasion of a situation that might seem a little bit more threatening I always realise what a good Muslim I actually am. Good not as far as my performance of religious ritual duties or my avoidance of sin is concerned, but good in my well-established fatalism. I remember one time being on a plane that, shortly after departure from Kuala Lumpur, was hit by lightning. Of course, conventional wisdom tells us that lightning only rarely actually affect aeroplanes. But this was a Malaysia Airlines flight in September 2014, shortly after two terrible tragedies, one MA flight that was accidentally shot down over Ukraine in July, and another that was (probably) intentionally crashed by a suicidal pilot over the Indian Ocean in August. After these tragedies many people became hesitant about flying with the airline. It had gained an undeserved unlucky reputation. But I had, nevertheless, specifically chosen to fly with Malaysia Airlines at that time. I have always considered them my favourite airline. I always loved their excellent food and their lovely entertainment programme, and their wonderfully friendly and helpful staff. When the lightning struck our flight I did, however, wonder for a few seconds whether I would now become part of a third tragedy striking the airline in that sad year. At that moment, none of us passengers knew that this was a lightning strike. We just felt a strong impact and our plane was shaking terribly and then falling for a few meters until it caught itself again. It then took a few minutes for the captain to inform the passengers that everything was alright. In that moment, when I felt the impact and the shaking and then the short fall downwards, I suddenly became incredibly calm and serene and I quietly said to myself, 'Oh, this is it now? It's time for you already? *La ilaha illallah*.'.

At the beginning of the Covid-19 pandemic, I often had to think of that moment. I have never been afraid of death but I have to admit that there have been times in my life when I had been afraid of dying. Whatever awaits us after the veils of existence are lifted from us does not scare me. But I do acknowledge that for many of us the process that precedes that moment can be a very unpleasant one, often marked by physical pain. That was certainly something that we also heard about in the experience of the people that were dying from Covid-19 infections in Italy during the early stages of the pandemic. The reports that reached us spoke of terrible pain. A feeling as if your lungs are filled with broken glass. And of the terrible loneliness of dying in isolation, without being able to receive visitors or to properly say good bye to your loved ones.

These were scary reports and we still read such stories from all over the world. These reports worried me incredibly. My mother was diagnosed with asthma in childhood, and with COPD (chronic obstructive pulmonary disease) in recent years, and respiratory infections tend to always hit her terribly. Twice I have seen her being put into an artificial coma because her lungs have not been able to process enough oxygen. The last time this happened the doctors had almost lost hope and our family had prepared itself for possible loss. Fortunately, she survived. I was diagnosed with asthma when I was young and probably have COPD as well (even though the diagnosis on that has been less clear). I perceive the pandemic first and foremost as a threat to my mother, and then also as a threat to myself.

When the news about people dying of Covid-19 first started filtering through to me, I couldn't help but constantly contemplate what it would be like if either my mother or myself would have to go through this ordeal. An indescribable feeling of horror. But then I remembered that moment on that strange flight and I thought, 'don`t worry, death will come eventually. Whatever pain and struggle there will be, in the end you will just feel calm and serene and welcome what will come'. This has not lifted my worries for my mother or other loved ones from me. But to some extent I do have the hope that death does not only come to me, but also to other people, like that.

I do wonder whether my recurring dreams about flying during this pandemic also have something to do with this knowledge. I do not dream about turbulence and I have never dreamed about that lightning strike. My dream journeys are always very comfortable and joyful right up to the moment I realise that I actually should not be on that flight because we are in the middle of a pandemic. But in *ta`bîr*, the classic Islamic art of dream interpretation, it is often assumed that the actual meaning of a dream is not to be found in its most obvious aspects. Rather, its meaning hides in its nooks and crannies, just as the meaning of the verses of the Qur'an or the meaning of a *ghazal* often does not reveal itself fully at first sight.

The obvious, the *zâhir* exegesis of my viral dreams is that I long for travels and journeys and that I want to escape this situation that restricts my ability to move across our beautiful globe. But hidden, the *bâtin*, hermeneutics (ta'wîl) of my dreams may teach me something else. They may whisper to me: sleep well, sleep tight, even when the world around you is shaking. Be serene, be calm, there is nothing to fear. The journey of this life continues, even if the road is rough.

EXISTENTIAL TERROR

James Brooks

For a year or so in my teens I was convinced that I – and almost everybody I knew – would die in a terrifying brain-disease epidemic. Sometimes this foreknowledge would sit quietly, emitting a faint unnerving hum, in the darker recesses of my psyche. But sometimes it would spring forth in epic uncontrollable tantrums, teeth bared and glistening with blood, to tear my inner world apart.

These tantrums could last for weeks before calming down, only to flare up again. Several nights I lay awake till the early morning, hot with fear, trying to snatch some hope, or at the very least meaning, from the fated carnage. More often though, the tantrums would peak in the daytime, forcing me into a curious double existence. I remember a school trip to the Houses of Parliament in late 1995 or early 1996. Outwardly, there I was on the bus, chipping in with the banter, laughing at jokes about teachers out of earshot, making additions to the absurd adolescent flights of fancy. Inwardly, however, I was lost in blind panic, unable to break or squash the unrelenting monologue. *They're all gonna die. You will too. See it. In a bed on thin dirty sheets. Mewling, shaking, drooling. And then nothingness, forever. As if you never existed. The void.*

As we made our way back home with the Thames on one side and the smartest bits of London on the other, I imagined the city as it would be once the epidemic had truly hit. The hospitals would have filled up with only one kind of patient – the kind that would never improve – and millions would be grieving and waiting for their turn to come. I imagined London as a hopeless, crumbling sanitorium.

I had not gone mad. People across the country were harbouring a pathogen which had laid low in their cells for years but was poised to eviscerate them at any moment. Soon enough I could watch the shaky home video footage of the epidemic's first victims as it played on the TV news, realising my worst fears. Meanwhile, harrowing reports from parents of their children's slide into incapacity filled newspaper columns.

From *The Independent*, 21 March 1996:

> The most frightening thing was the similarity between his condition and disease we have seen cows suffering from. It included shaking, nervousness and what appeared to be hallucinations,' [Derek] Hall said [of his son Peter]. 'In 12 months we saw him deteriorate into someone who could not walk, talk or do anything for himself.

The brain-disease epidemic I feared was that brought about by 'mad cow disease', or to use its proper name, bovine spongiform encephalopathy (BSE). When the story of a new disease sweeping through British cattle broke in Autumn 1987, I was nine: old enough to watch the reports on the BBC Six O'Clock News. Images of cattle foaming at the mouth, trembling and sliding their way across cowshed floors were followed by ministers glibly relating that there was 'no evidence that this disease could infect humans', perhaps before intoning the government mantra 'beef is safe'.

The pattern of frightening revelations and horror-film imagery followed by government denial played out in irregular instalments on our living-room TV for the following nine years. As evidence leaked out that BSE had crossed the species barrier into lab animals – cue clip of albino mice in crowded plastic boxes – the government rebuttals only grew in fervour. The government had ordered all cattle showing signs of BSE to be slaughtered in June 1988 – cue swollen cattle entering incinerators – but by then an estimated one million infected cattle had already entered the human food chain. Scientists expected there to be a decades-long asymptomatic incubation period after infection. The UK was sitting on a timebomb of terminal illness.

I do not remember what, if anything, provoked it, but sometime in mid-1995, roughly when I turned seventeen, my brain seized on the BSE crisis and wouldn't let go. When on 20 March 1996, the government succumbed to reality and admitted a 'probable link' between BSE and a new brain disease which had already claimed a handful of lives, I flipped. We were at the bottom of the curve, I thought. Soon enough it would rise like a great wave, engulfing everything I knew. I could see it coming.

BSE and its human version, variant Creutzfeldt-Jakob Disease (vCJD), are not caused by a virus but a tiny speck of misfolded protein called a prion. And yet, long incubation period aside, vCJD looks more like the kind of deadly virus that runs amok in Hollywood movies than almost all genuine viral diseases. For one, patients are zombified, even taking on a slow, shuffling gait before becoming bed-bound. For another, just as in zombie movies – most of which imagine a virus as the causative pathogen – vCJD can be transferred in a drop of blood. This is why anybody who lived in the UK between 1980 and 1996 is banned from giving blood anywhere else in the world. But vCJD most obviously resembles the doomsday virus of screenwriters' dreams in one chilling detail – it carries a one hundred per cent death rate.

Appropriately, a Hollywood movie about an apocalyptic viral pandemic rescued my sanity. It showed me that my overweening paranoia was being fed largely by my subconscious dealings with the deepest taboo in Western consumerist society. A taboo which rises closest to the surface whenever viruses appear on screen. Death. Of course, death.

12 Monkeys was released in UK cinemas exactly one month after the government dropped its 'probable link' bombshell. The film opens with green capped-up typewriter lettering tapped out on a black screen. As I read it, I felt a rush of recognition, as if, finally, something would deal with what was really going on in the world, and in my head. The green lettering read:

> '...5 BILLION PEOPLE WILL DIE FROM A DEADLY VIRUS IN 1997...
> ...THE SURVIVORS WILL ABANDON THE SURFACE OF THE PLANET...
> ...ONCE AGAIN THE ANIMALS WILL RULE THE WORLD...'
>
> Excerpts from interview with clinically diagnosed paranoid schizophrenic, April 12, 1990 – Baltimore County Hospital

The 'paranoid schizophrenic' in question is the lead character, with whom I share a first name: James Cole. *12 Monkeys* occasionally flirts with the idea that his diagnosis may be correct, and everything he speaks of – and much of what we see – is psychotic fabrication. But it mostly takes the line that Cole is in fact a time-traveller from the year 2035 who has been sent back in time to locate the origin of the virus which will destroy humanity. Once Cole has located it, a scientist will make the journey across time to study the virus 'in its pure form, before it mutates', as he says at one point, in the hope of finding a cure.

One of the film's many triumphs lies in how it enables suspension of disbelief in Cole's apparently ludicrous backstory. It does this by forgoing nearly all the clichés of the sci-fi genre. In the film's version of 2035, there are no kitsch costumes, no infallible space-age technology that responds seamlessly to its operator's will, and no Shakespearean actors intoning incomprehensible fantasy-world babble. Instead the future world is a junkyard version of the present. This is exactly in keeping with the aesthetic sensibilities of its director, Terry Gilliam, and what you could reasonably expect if humans had been forced to set up underground in a hurry. Technology in 2035 is also suitably cranky and the scientists who run it less than masterful. 'Science ain't an exact science with these clowns,' Cole is told after he returns from his first time-trip, which mistakenly drops him in 1990 rather than his target date of 1996.

The film uses a linear model of time so that when Cole heads back to the past it is to *his* past, not one in some alternate dimension. In other words, from the vantage of 2035, everything that Cole does in 1990 or 1996 – or, again accidentally, 1917 – has already happened. Cole is therefore a fated character, as in Greek tragedy, who exists in a permanent state of unfreedom. He starts the film as a convict who is 'volunteered' into the time-travel mission and then, once he arrives in 1990, is immediately arrested and locked in a holding cell before being sent to a secure asylum. He spends the second reel on the run from the police while the panel of scientists from 2035 who give him his orders track him via a device in his teeth. Cole is not his own man.

In a performance that stands in stark contrast to his displays of testosterone-fuelled bravado in the *Die Hard* franchise, Bruce Willis plays Cole as someone profoundly vulnerable, without an ego, almost without any discernible character. It is no accident that he is called different names by the film's main characters. He is 'Cole' for the panel of scientists, 'Bob' (my father's name, incidentally) for a mysterious voice he hears at crucial junctures, and briefly 'Arnold Pettibone' for Brad Pitt's character, Jeffrey Goines, the man who may or may not be responsible for unleashing the virus. Only Cole's psychiatrist, kidnap victim and eventual co-conspirator

Kathryn Railly – played superbly by Madeleine Stowe – calls him 'James'. Multiple suspicious protagonists trying to push an identity on a bewildered lead character, while only a stunningly beautiful woman accepts that person as they are, is a set-up that will resonate powerfully with a teenage boy.

The assonances with my personal BSE-related psychodrama were even more compelling. BSE was a product of mankind's abusive relationship with nature. It was created by feeding cows the ground-up brains of sheep that had contracted a similar neurodegenerative condition called scrapie. It spread when the ground-up brains of BSE-infected cows were fed to other cows. At one point during his trip to 1990, Cole sits in the day room of the asylum watching a report on animal experimentation on TV. He watches rabbits being constrained, struggling, and injected with who-knows-what. He whispers disgustedly: 'Maybe the human race deserves to be wiped out.' At the time, I found it hard to disagree.

Cole's status as a seer, as an isolated carrier of terrible knowledge about the future, resonated with me profoundly. His predicament is inadvertently summarised by Railly, whose academic interest is the apocalyptic visions of psychotics. Giving a lecture shortly before she is kidnapped by Cole in 1996 (he was her patient during his accidental stay in 1990) Railly speaks of such visionaries suffering

> a self-inflicted agony we call the 'Cassandra complex'. Cassandra, in Greek legend, was condemned to know the future but to be disbelieved when she foretold it. Hence, the agony of foreknowledge combined with the impotence to do anything about it.

Cole himself puts it more bluntly. In one of relatively few action scenes for a time-travel adventure movie, Cole beats a pair of gangsters to death in a derelict theatre after they have attacked him and Railly. Feeling for the pulse of one, Railly yells: 'Oh, Jesus! James, you killed him!' In his desperate, spent voice, Cole returns: 'All I see are dead people.'

That is precisely where I was with vCJD in April 1996. All I saw were dead people: unknowing incubators of a lethal pathogen, most of them oblivious to the disaster that would befall them. I didn't talk about my fears that much, but whenever I did, those who I spoke to were largely unconcerned. I remember sitting across the school lunch table from my best friend, and him telling me that as long as he got three years of partying at university in, he wasn't too worried about what came after. Sorry, what? There was no reason to believe we hadn't all eaten diseased meat and were harbouring microscopic particles that would eat holes in our brains and kill us. And you're not too worried about that, no?

Indeed, *12 Monkeys* deals with the universal Cassandra complex – the agony and impotence arising from foreknowledge of our inescapable mortality. It is a film where the principal story relates to Cole's status as a man who, when he was a child, literally witnessed his own death. In a universally relatable move, Cole buried this foreknowledge within his subconscious only for it to haunt the rest of his life.

Like Cole, but somewhat more metaphorically, I also witnessed my death at an early age. Once every school holiday, my mother would take me on the forty-mile train ride into London, to visit one tourist attraction and browse the huge department stores. When I was about eight, we visited the London Planetarium, a circular auditorium beneath a giant dome that served as a projection screen for shows about space and astronomy. We watched a show in which the entire history of the universe, starting with the big bang and ending with a discussion of how it would end: the big rip or the big freeze or the big crunch. I was soon seized by a terror like nothing I had felt before. I did not come from a religious home but my parents had sent me to a Church of England school and inadvertently uncovered a prodigious propensity for religious faith. I was a fervent believer, voluntarily attending school Bible club with the children of good Christian families. Now, sitting panicked in the auditorium watching the Earth being cooked and eaten by the sun, I wondered where Jesus was in this story. Where was God? Humanity's place within the universe was not even worth mentioning and mine even less so. It would be over as soon as it began. We were all on the slide to oblivion. I wanted to know: why wasn't everybody screaming?

If there are comical overtones to this scene, I didn't feel them at the time. I later learnt, though, that my experience was akin to that assigned to victims of the Total Perspective Vortex, a device from *The Restaurant at the End of the Universe*, the second of Douglas Adams' comedic science fiction novels in the *Hitchhiker's Guide to the Galaxy* series. The vortex is an execution device that gives those who enter it

> just one momentary glimpse of the entire unimaginable infinity of creation, and somewhere in it a tiny little marker, a microscopic dot on a microscopic dot, which says: 'You are here.'

This is enough to induce such a rush of such cosmic horror in subjects that they drop dead. As Adams says, 'if life is going to exist in a universe of this size, then the one thing it cannot afford to have is a sense of proportion.'

This paralysing vision of the futility of life, of the futility of *my* life and its imminent termination, persisted for months. It was my first, and by no means last, taste of what is called existential terror, or death anxiety. I say 'what is called' because I know that many people have never tasted it. For those people – the seventeenth century mathematician and thinker Blaise Pascal called you 'monsters', by the way – I am afraid I am unable to do justice to the full gripping horror of it. For me, the train of thought usually runs counter to that which occurred in my Planetarium episode. It normally starts with a creeping realisation of the absolute certainty that one day I will cease to exist. I become aware of what the late Philip Larkin – in his immaculate poem on the subject, *Aubade* – called

> The sure extinction that we travel to
> And shall be lost in always. Not to be here,
> Not to be anywhere,
> And soon; nothing more terrible, nothing more true.

From there, over the course of days, weeks, sometimes months, my mind races on a desperate journey into the future, sometimes even scrabbling about at the ends of the universe – the big rip, the big freeze, the big crunch, or whatever – to try and find some infinitesimal part of me, or just humanity, that will survive the end of time. Of course, I never find it, and I'm back to square one contemplating my own imminent annihilation. 'This is a special way of being afraid / No trick dispels', as the following lines of *Aubade* put it.

In its modern, medicalised 'mental health' configuration, psychology no longer addresses the possibility that some forms of psychic anguish are inherent in the human condition. It therefore has almost nothing to say about existential terror, mankind's inner reckoning with its ultimate fate.

But things were not always this way. In the 1950s and 1960s the existential school of psychology flourished, with its sights set squarely on the painful confrontation with the pre-existing conditions of human existence, or what Sigmund Freud called the reality principle. When existential psychologists strayed from the individual ramifications of this confrontation and into the social, they stressed the great and destructive forces that could be unleashed. It is no coincidence that nearly all the leading existential psychologists were Jewish – often, like Erich Fromm, people who had fled the Holocaust or, like Viktor Frankl, death-camp survivors. We should note in passing that while the cataclysms of the Second World War may have inspired reflection on the deep-seated reasons for human destructiveness among thinkers in the West, those brought about by colonialism did no such thing.

Ernest Becker was Jewish and had helped liberate the Nazi concentration camps during the war. He was an anthropologist rather than a psychologist but he drew heavily on existential psychology to produce his magnum opus *The Denial of Death*, published, with grim irony, in late 1973, just three months before he died. Like many texts of existential psychology, *The Denial of Death* is in large part an exercise in dissent from Freudian orthodoxy. In particular, Becker sought to overthrow the libido as the primal source of psychic energy motivating human behaviour and replace it with, yes, the need to deny our mortality.

Becker's argument, paraphrased quite freely, runs like this. Humans are the only species of animal cursed with the Cassandra complex that comes from knowing we will one day be consigned to nothingness. This knowledge is intolerable to us and causes us to suffer paralysing existential terror whenever it is apprehended. No trick can dispel this fear (Larkin was right) and we are reminded daily of our mortality by our bodies, those compacted clods of dust, which to dust shall be returned (Genesis 3:19). Our only escape from this impossible predicament lies in creating a life in a socially constructed symbolic world tethered to but distinct from the physical one. The symbolic world is the repository of all the meanings we attach to the events that happen in the physical world that are, in themselves, entirely meaningless. Whereas we are sure to be annihilated in the physical world, in the symbolic realm we can commit to an 'immortality project' which, we imagine, will outlast our earthly expiration. Our immortality project may take the form of dissolution into what people often refer to as 'something bigger than yourself', be it a mass cultural construct like religion or nationalism, or a more intimate commitment to family and community. To put all this another way, human culture is an elaborate, symbolic defence mechanism against the knowledge of death.

Becker's thesis may look untestable. It is not. Since the mid-1980s, three US psychologists – Jeff Greenberg, Sheldon Solomon and Tom Pyszczynski – have dedicated themselves to picking it apart and testing its experimental validity. Out of these experiments grew terror management theory, a psychological paradigm that posits the need to avoid or buffer death anxiety as a critical driver of human thought and behaviour, much as Becker predicted. One of the trio's crucial discoveries from their experiments was the extent to which people's commitment to their cultural worldviews – to their immortality projects, in other words – can be heightened by even the slightest reminders of death. They also discovered that exposure to different cultural worldviews held by others provoked the same effect. It would appear that contact with other worldviews and religious beliefs – that is, other, often incompatible, immortality projects – causes us to subconsciously question our own. It provokes a degree of cognitive dissonance which we seek to diffuse by clinging ever tighter to *our* views and cultural identities. This all has profound ramifications in a modern world increasingly immersed in decontextualised onscreen depictions of death and calamity, be they real or fictitious, and the never-ending battles of competing worldviews in the 'culture wars'. These constant mortality reminders will only work to harden and radicalise people in their views and make finding common ground ever harder.

For the irreligious, the experiments on cultural attachment that led Greenberg, Solomon and Pyszczynski to their conclusions can sound amusingly subversive. In one, two groups of non-observant American students from secular or mildly Christian family backgrounds were given basic personality questionnaires to fill, with one group's forms including subtle reminders of death within the questions. Then the students were led to a room where they were asked to hang a crucifix on a wall, but found only the crucifix and a nail waiting for them on the desk. Those students who had been reminded of their mortality took on average twice as long as those who hadn't to complete the task. They often tried futile alternative strategies before bowing to the inevitable and using the crucifix to hammer the nail into the chipboard.

Certainly, Becker would have agreed with Larkin's assessment of religion in *Aubade* as 'That vast moth-eaten musical brocade / Created to pretend we never die'. Nevertheless, that remark has lost its pertinence in the contemporary West where religion is in decline (Northern Europe) or had its ideology twisted beyond recognition by consumerist individualism (the US). It is also the case that the collapse of this death-denying cultural framework across much of the West has not led to a more mature societal reckoning with death. Nothing could be further from the truth. As palliative care researchers Liz Grant, Scott Murray and Aziz Sheikh pointed out in an accessible and profound paper in the BMJ in 2010:

> Death and dying were keystones of the grand narrative of religion. But religions, in Western cultures, are disappearing, and grand narratives have been replaced by worldviews driven by individual success that are not so much death denying as blind to death.

In social and psychological terms, this cultural turn away from sense-making about death has been counterproductive. Whether we like it or not, death itself is still with us, is still a human universal, and we need a buffer to help us deal with it. As William James, the American philosopher and psychologist, wrote in 1902, in a passage quoted in *The Denial of Death*:

> Let sanguine healthy-mindedness do its best with its strange power of living in the moment and ignoring and forgetting, still the evil background is really there to be thought of, and the skull will grin in at the banquet.

More than that, no longer covered by the moth-eaten brocade, the skull appears more lurid, its grimace more appalling, and is free to unleash 'a great variety of morbid symptoms', to borrow Antonio Gramsci's famous phrase, in our culture. If you doubt this, just go and watch a big-budget Hollywood movie.

As Theodor Adorno once said about Hollywood: 'the dream does not dream'. That is, although popular American cinema appears to offer escape from capitalism's cultural neuroses, it in fact reflects and reinforces them. In this case, have you ever wondered why so many Hollywood films feature far-fetched, overblown life-or-death scenarios for the lead characters? Or why these films sacrifice all plot to a naked battle for survival? Or how so many of us in the prosperous West, where life is easiest and longest lasting, can relate to such stories? Now you have your answer. Hollywood movies are often no more than noisy and graphic sublimations of our death anxiety – the skull grinning in at the banquet.

While this is true of almost all blockbusters that aren't romcoms, it's glaringly so for any film from the last 25 years with the word 'virus' in its plot summary. This is probably because viruses offer screenwriters a device where death can literally spread like a plague, striking down anyone and everyone. *Resident Evil*, *28 Days Later,* even *Contagion*, which attempted a degree of realism, can all be read as exercises in sublimating consumer culture's deep existential terror. But perhaps the most florid outburst of death anxiety to ever appear on screen is *World War Z*, a 2013 film about a near extinction-level viral pandemic that features Brad Pitt and David Morse, two actors who had pivotal roles in *12 Monkeys*.

The similarities end there. Whereas *12 Monkeys* is a film that develops its complex plot and themes with care, subtly dropping clues to allow the audience to follow, *World War Z* is mostly Brad Pitt escaping death in a series of ridiculous action-film sequences – running through machine-gun spray, crawling out of plane crashes, jumping onto other planes as cities collapse behind him. The film could hardly be any less subtle if it flashed up title cards every five minutes saying: 'MEN! LOOK AT MUSCLY BRAD PITT FULFILLING YOUR WILDEST DEATH-DENIAL FANTASIES! BRAD PITT WILL NEVER DIE! IDENTIFY WITH HIM!' I guess women are supposed to identify with Pitt's onscreen wife (Mireille Enos) who spends much of her screen time crying over Pitt being off saving the world while lovingly caring for their shared immortality projects. I mean children.

We know we're in for one long draining exposition of death anxiety about ten minutes into the film when Pitt – his character is called Gerry Lane, but nobody who has seen this film will remember that – is stuck in traffic with his family. There's some commotion up ahead and we understand what's going on when an army of zombies comes stampeding through. We see people pulled from their cars and bitten, before suffering violent convulsions and transforming into ravenous crater-eyed cadavers. Having the first onscreen outbreak occur while Pitt is stationary in the people-carrier with his wife and kids is an obvious stab at suburban-dad identification but the filmmakers also hit on something deeper. Nothing is more likely to induce reflection on the absurdity and futility of existence than being stuck in a traffic jam. Talking Heads' frontman David Byrne warned us about being behind the wheel in 'Once in a Lifetime', the group's defining single. I'm sure many of us have felt our graves open up beneath us as exhaust fumes rise in plumes from the car in front and the kids squabble in the back seat.

At several points *World War Z* is little more than an audio-visual display of the utter terror unleashed by the idea of death untrammelled by religion. In many religious traditions the dead watch over us, they are our ancestors who guide us, maybe they rest in eternal peace, at one with the divine. Here the dead are crazed animated corpses that seek only to sink their rotten teeth into your flesh and bring you down to their wretched state. Several of the scenes in the film are reminiscent of the gruesome hellscapes of Hieronymus Bosch. In one, the zombies clamber over each other in a great mountain of bodies to scale a huge wall protecting Jerusalem. (Yes, I saw a particularly foul parallel there, too, and wasn't reassured of it being an unfortunate coincidence when the film started fêting Mossad.)

I do wonder how things would have been different for me had *World War Z* come out in 1996, rather than *12 Monkeys*, and I'd gone along to see it. Such a barrage of apocalyptic imagery might have pushed me over the edge. Instead, the fact that *12 Monkeys* was not really about a doomsday virus but about Cole, a man who had witnessed his own death, helped awaken me from my mad-cow nightmare. I could see that my visions of a zombie apocalypse were just my personal death anxiety run riot. I understood that I wasn't really scared of a vCJD epidemic. I was scared of death.

The great wave of vCJD cases never came. Deaths from the disease peaked in 2000 and to date one hundred seventy-eight people in the UK have died from it, with no deaths reported in the last four years. Worryingly, there is good reason to suspect there will be a second wave of deaths, maybe two or three decades from now, of people whose genetic make-up means they harbour the prion for longer. But it seems impossible that vCJD will fell millions, as I had imagined. It's worth noting that my fear of an apocalyptic epidemic was not irrational, it's more that my weakly repressed death anxiety had pushed me to believe – to *want* to believe, in a way – the very worst-case scenario. Having to deal with mortality alone, without a cultural framework to rely on, produces 'a great variety of morbid symptoms' in people, as I say. Catastrophism is one of mine.

In April 1996, after watching *12 Monkeys*, I started to lose interest in mad cow disease. I had other things on my mind. I managed to scrape the necessary A-level grades and gained a place at university. After eighteen years stuck in the stultifying, alienated atmosphere of the provincial suburbs, I was going to London, where everything happened. I left and never looked back.

Still, attacks of existential terror have hit me at irregular intervals ever since. For years, I wished for a trick that would dispel them, but no longer. For one thing, I now appreciate what they give me: an appreciation that, yes, all *is* vanity. So many people are locked into an absurd struggle to achieve significance in the symbolic realm, to counter their imminent extinction in the physical one. In the social milieu in which I now exist – middle-class North London – such symbolic heroism (as Becker called it) centres on achieving and maintaining social status by furthering one's career and adopting a kind of 'reasonable', centrist, cosmopolitan political outlook. It looks silly to me, and I'm glad I don't waste my time playing along with it. But there's something else, too. I've accepted that my bouts of existential terror are a sign that I'm not really living, that I'm just going through the motions. They are thus a spur for change and growth.

I often think of a passage by Primo Levi, the writer and chemist who spent eleven months of his life in the Auschwitz III concentration camp, or 'the Lager' as he referred to it in his writings (keeping the German word). Evidently, this was a place where blindness to death was impossible. In *The Drowned and the Saved*, Levi talks of how, under such conditions, believers of any religion or political creed fared better. They held on to

> a millennial tomorrow so that there might be a sense of sacrificing themselves, a place in heaven or on earth where justice and compassion had won, or would win in a perhaps remote but certain future.

This, of course, is their immortality project. Non-believers did not have such a wellspring of hope to draw on. For them, being confronted with the inevitability of death led them to fixate on it. Levi cites the Auschwitz survivor Jean Améry who wrote of so much talk in the camp centring on how it might be best to die. But Levi, a non-believer, managed to resist death colonising his mind.

> Perhaps because I was younger, perhaps because I was more ignorant than [Améry], or less marked, or less conscious, I almost never had the time to devote to death. I had many other things to keep me busy – find a bit of bread, avoid exhausting work, patch my shoes, steal a broom, or interpret the signs and faces around me.

And then these words, that everyone should know:

> The aims of life are the best defence against death: and not only in the Lager.

ARTS AND LETTERS

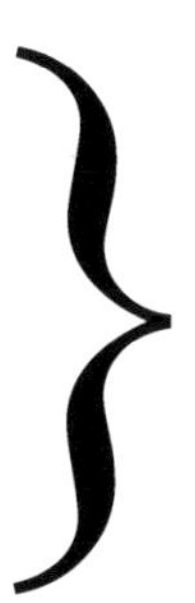

SHORT STORY

RECREATION

Uzmah Ali

From behind my plastic wall, I hear the hollow footsteps of Munro. Munro always comes in at daybreak, as is her habit. A Munro day always fills me with dread. But it's also a two day marker; only two days until Higgins starts his shift. And his shifts are always much more bearable.

Munro's footsteps stop just outside of the door, and I can hear her punch the numbers into the keypad, and the pistons on the door hiss as they loosen. Then the tinny jangling of keys, and the soft clicking of the lock, the turning of the handle. Then she opens the door, and comes in.

Munro, is an older lady. I only know she's older, because she leaves magazines near my wall for me to look at. Almost always they're fashion magazines, glossy and bright, with images of thin tanned women in what I think looks like underwear, but are actually clothes for swimming, Munro tells me. They all have smooth skin in a way that Munro doesn't. I pointed this out to her once, and she got really angry. I wasn't quite sure what I had done, but she shouted at me, and told me to mind my own business. I told Higgins about it, on a Higgins day. He said that some women didn't like to be reminded that they weren't young anymore, and it wasn't polite to remind them.

I thought that was stupid. Everyone's going to grow old, and there's no way to stop it.

Smiles, sand, and blue sky and water. Those are the pictures in the magazines. That's called outside. Of course, I know that if I ever went outside people would scream, and run away from me. If they came too close to me, they would die. I'm the last contagion, says Munro. That's why it's better that I'm in the plastic room.

Because of people like me, there was a war, and killing and a pandemic. Most of us had been hunted down and killed. But, my mother, also hunted down and killed so Higgins told me, gave birth to me before they got her. And someone took pity on this poor baby – that was me - and some scientists with immunity decided to raise her in a lab. And there was no one left in the world with the living contagion, apart from me. So it was up to the scientists to raise me away from everyone else, and do experiments and whatever the hell else they needed to do, to find a cure to this disease that killed two billion people.

And there were only eight billion people on the planet before the catastrophe. Because of people like me one in four died. That's what Higgins told me, anyway.

So, I'm stuck in the plastic room, until I die I suppose. But for the safety of others as I'm constantly told by Munro. At least I'm fed, and Munro and Higgins look after me. They've fed me, taught me stuff, and also, Higgins'll get kids in from the nearby village, and they'll play chess or cards with me through the plastic wall. It's just that they need to move the pieces for me. And that's not so bad, at least I have someone my age to hang out with.

They talk about stuff which makes me a bit sad though sometimes, like school and friends and stuff. I don't know what any of this means. But if they let me go, people will die. Too bad I suppose.

'How's my favourite experimental subject today? Isn't she lucky to get another day in paradise! Get showered, then I need to sedate you,'

There's a little windowless bathroom round the back of the plastic room. Somewhere, where I can have some privacy, get showered and other stuff. It's monitored on the screens. Whenever I go and get showered, Higgins always asks me in a really gentle way, and puts his paper over the monitor, so I know he's not looking at me as I wash. Munro, on the other hand, seems to think that I'm a specimen, and my body is her property, so will watch me as I shower. She likes to survey me for science, so she says.

I go into the bathroom. As soon as I open the door the lights flick on, and the bassy purr of the extractor fan begins. I don't get any of the fancy soap that they have in Munro's magazines. I get the only soap I've ever known, with a smell I'm used to, a smell partway between the crayons I'm sometimes allowed to draw with, and the toothpaste they leave me with. The water is the same temperature that I left it yesterday, just a bit warmer than my skin. When I'm feeling more penned in than usual, I'll put the water on really hot. In a way the scorching feeling, the way I need to grit my teeth under scalding water gives me something to feel.

I take a quick perfunctory shower. This is a Munro shower, where I know she's watching me get showered as I sip my morning coffee, and not a Higgins shower, where he walks away from the monitor to make sure I can bathe in confidence. I've tested this. There's been times where I've thrown suds onto the little camera, the only black thing in the room against the blue eggshell. On a Munro day, she'll tell me to *rinse the camera immediately.* Whereas if I throw suds on the camera on a Higgins day, he'll say nothing. And when I emerge from the bathroom, he'll be at the far side of the lab, away from the bathroom monitor. He likes to give me my privacy like that.

Shower, brush teeth. I'm hoping by the time I've got showered, my breakfast would've been deposited in the lobby. The lobby is the little cubbyhole which is used to exchange things. Although the only scientists allowed in the lab are those that have developed immunity, I'm told that things can only be handed to me through the cubbyhole. The less physical human contact I have the better. Reduces the chance of cross-contamination. I don't think I've been hugged since I was three. When I was really little, the people who would tend to me would be wearing full radiation suits. Actually, my first memory, is standing at the edge of a crib screaming for attention, and someone in an orange suit, coming over, smiling at me, and putting a bottle in my mouth. The people who nursed and nurtured me are still in the facility, so I've been told, and they sometimes drop by to say hi.

I walk out of the bathroom, into the cubbyhole-lobby, which is another windowless room with fluorescent lights that flick on as soon as you open the door. I'm only a couple of sidesteps from the plastic room. The room where everyone can see me. Once, Munro left a magazine called 'Interiors' near my plastic wall. I looked at it for hours. The 'living room' on the front cover looked so inviting. Dark green throws, tall lamps with soft lighting, some nice curtains on the window. Maybe I'll get to live somewhere like that when they're done experimenting on me.

There a neatly folded pile of clothes in the cubbyhole, a white cotton smock, underwear, a cardigan and a towel. I towel dry my hair, and put on the clothes.

I emerge into the plastic room, and wait for Munro. She'll tell me what we're doing today. With Higgins, it's a mix of learning stuff, chatting, 'craft activities' which I'm actually getting a bit bored of, and think I might be getting a bit too old for them. But he's kinder than Munro, and that's why I look forward to the Higgins days.

'CF23 – you're looking a bit chubby. Are you due your period?'

'Don't know, thought you'd know better than me,' I say, with an indifferent tone. I suspect I don't look fat at all. I suspect Munro is just trying to add some spice to her day.

I take my breakfast tray to the pillows in the corner of the plastic room, and sit down on the floor cushions. The cushions are stained and lumpy, donations from Higgin's wife. But at least they're mine, and soft, unlike the other bits of furniture in the plastic room. The plastic room has a plastic wall through which the lab is visible. The scientists can sometimes do this thing where the plastic wall becomes black, and then they watch me. One way mirror it's called. They usually do this when they've given me some task to perform. Munro prefers not to use the one way mirror. She likes to know everything that's going on in my world.

'Don't eat!' Munro squawks as I reach for the bread on my tray, 'I need to take your fasting bloods today,'

It'll definitely be a specimen day today, I think to myself. A specimen day is when I'm more specimen than human. And they are almost always with Munro.

She puts her hands through the gloves that are attached to the plastic wall that hang there like lifeless, dying daffodils, most of the time, until one of the scientists decides that they want to prod me. Of course, they could unlock the plastic room, put on a radiation suit and come in. But that would be too humanising, and therefore, it's against protocol.

'Come on, I haven't got all day, over here,' snaps Munro, her tired skin puckering into a sweep of minor rage, and her coarse mousey brown hair falling into her eyes.

I follow the drill and walk over to the rubber marigolds, that look like ravenous tropical crabs from the nature documentaries that Higgins has shown me. Munro has the extractors in her fingertips, and I wait for vibration to move through the gloves, into my skin, so she can remove as much blood or plasma, or whatever it is she wants. The feeling always shocks me a little, like a searing heat moving through all of my bones. There'll be yellowy aching blisters all over my wrists after this, and they'll take days to heal.

I feel my knees begin to buckle below me, and I want to hit Munro, but the energy is seeping away from me and my eyelids are beginning to slide over my eyes. Higgins always asks whether or not he can sedate me. Munro just does it.

When I come to, my smock is raised to my waist and there is a searing all the way from my waist to me feet. Munro has probably done some of her weird experiments again; the ones where she'll come into the plastic room in her anti-contagion suit and throw me around like a rag doll while I'm semi-conscious. I can't wait for a Higgins day.

Just one more day.

The next day passes much like the first. Only this time, it appears that Munro is beginning to lose her ability to sedate me in a measured way. This time, it feels like I'm completely out for the count after about three seconds. Higgins has warned against this type of sedation; he says it's dangerous for my heart. But all Munro can see is the contagion seeping through my skin and breath and tears. I'm deathly dangerous. I wonder what it would be like to be born free, but I know myself too well now. If I start thinking these thoughts, I'll stop washing, I'll stop eating, and I'll start looking for things to cut my skin with. I'm a survivor. No matter how hard Munro tries, she can't infiltrate my mind. My thoughts are my own, and I will continue to think like a calm, kind, rational person, and have a private space within myself, that I allow to hate Munro, without ever letting on.

The sedation that Munro had given me was so strong that I don't wake until mid-afternoon. I'm usually woken at eight o'clock, but this time I wake up at around eleven. And I'm so glad to see Higgins. His greying hair and back are hunched over some machines when I opened my eyes. I have enough strength to push myself up, and sat with my knees hunched to my chest.

Higgins turned around, he must have heard some rustling. A smile emerges across his face.

'Hello you! I tried to wake you, but you looked like you needed the sleep,'

'Professor Munro sedated me. It was much stronger than usual,'

'How strange, we hadn't planned any experiments where sedation would be necessary,'

'Well, you know she likes to see me suffer. Either that, or she likes to shut me up,'

'Don't talk about Professor Munro like that,' said Higgins 'She's looked after you since you were an infant,'

I stared straight ahead. I knew if I answered Higgins back, my voice would be full of tears.

Professor Higgins, appearing to sense how upset I was, quickly changed the subject.

'So, I have a schedule for you today. I think Professor Munro has taken enough blood from you to keep me busy for most of the day. So no prodding or extractions today. But after you get showered, I can get you a late breakfast, and put on one of those nature documentaries that you like. How does that sound?'

I smiled back at Higgins, and he tapped softly on my plastic wall, the way he always showed affection.

'My wife has got some blankets that she crocheted a few years back, and she was going to send them to the charity shop. I said that I'd bring them here and let you have the first look at them. Something to make your plastic room feel a bit homely,'

I was so touched that I walk quickly into my bathroom and wipe away my tears. There was a reason I looked forward to Higgins days.

When I was done, there was a tray of bread, cheese and pastries in my cubby, which I took to the plastic room. Higgins had wheeled the television to near my wall. I tapped on the wall, and Higgins' head lifted from his work bench. He walked over and switched it on.

A man with a voice that sounded like an older man, a bit like Higgins I suppose, talks over snow-scapes in the arctic to soothing music. I could have listened to him for hours. There are pictures of penguins, and seal, and whales. I liked the pictures of shoals of fish under water the most. There are so many of them, moving in whatever direction they liked, free in vast expanses of frozen sea. Watching them float through the sea, made me feel like I was falling into some sort of trance.

Professor Higgins lets me watch two episodes, and then switches the television off. I wanted to cry, but I swallow my tears. Higgins comes to speak to me now, as is his habit.

'Did you enjoy the programme?'

'I want to watch it again,'

'Two hours is more than enough,'

I didn't realise it, but I must have been really upset and angry, because two hot tears rolled down my cheeks. I dip my face, embarrassed, not wanting Higgins to see.

'What's wrong?'

'It's just that sometimes I get sick of being in this room. I want to leave, I want to see people, I want to live!' I scream as I thump my hand against the plastic wall.

I fall onto the floor and sob and sob and sob.

Professor Higgins strokes the plastic wall between us, and looks a little sad.

He walks over to the machines in the far end of the lab and starts tinkering away, as if he's ignoring me.

The next day passes like every other, although Higgins is kind enough to get some puzzle books and pencils for me, and he lets me choose one of his old blankets.

Before he leaves he comes over to the plastic wall and pauses.

'I often take you for granted, CF23,'

I look at him. I don't know what he means, and it is strange for him to start such a deep conversation just before he leaves.

'Perhaps I'll die in the night, perhaps I won't be here in the morning. How would that make you feel?'

'Sad. Very sad. You've been so kind to me. I just wish I wasn't trapped all the time.'

'Well, I hope we do meet again,'

I shrug and wrinkle my forehead. I don't understand why he is being so cryptic.

'Um, I'm sure we will, stop being weird,'

'Wouldn't it be strange, if you could just push down the door handle of your room, and walk out tomorrow, unhindered,'

'But I don't want to cause the death of thousands. That's what you always said would happen if I left. Thousands and thousands of people would die of the virus, or there would be a war or something,'

Higgins quickly moved to one of the lab benches, like he had forgotten one of the experiments he was working on. He made some sort of muffled sound, he sometimes made that sound when he had a head-cold.

The sun rose the next day over the lab, and started creeping across the floor. I woke before my alarm, and bleary eyed I went into my bathroom to get showered. The lab clock said it was 7.35am, so it was twenty five minutes until Higgins was due to come in.

I always looked forward to a Higgins day.

By 8.45, I was hungry and Higgins was late. The latest he had ever been was ten minutes. I was beginning to worry. Two days Higgins, two days Munroe, two days Higgins, two days Munro. This was the rhythm I had known as far as I could remember. Occasionally both of them would come into the lab, and sometimes with the odd lab assistant. But for none to be here, near 9.00am was weird.

The day passes with not so much as a noise outside. I'm hungry and thirsty. No-one had even come in with a tray of food for my cubby. Nothing. I go over to the door in the corner of my plastic room and bang on it and scream. I shake the door handle, and it comes loose. I slide the door open. The only time I had ever seen this door open was when I've been sedated, and my eyes were about to close, and someone is about to take some part of me while they're wearing a radiation suit.

I sit in the doorway and stared ahead. I should have just shuffled my way out of the doorway, but I can barely move. I'm frozen.

Then I feel like I'm falling into some sort of unreality. I become frenzied, I decide I need to escape. I put on my shoes, and pushed the lab door open. Someone has forgotten to lock the door, and I push it open.

I expected a long corridor, like the corridors I had seen on the television, in the movies that Higgins let me watch sometime. The corridor is much shorter, and has a wooden door near the end of it.

I push the door open, and there is a gush of cold cold air, and a bit of wetness. Rain. I knew about rain because Higgins taught me about it. In this moment I realise I can't leave, I can't survive without Higgins or Munro or anything else. I don't know the world outside.

Then a woman runs up to me, quickly, and I look around. I see ambulances, and a few people dressed up like scientists.

Then I scream the loudest I ever scream in my life. The woman slows down, and walks up to me slowly.

I can barely breathe....*the virus...the virus...the virus.* The only words that are coming out of my mouth.

'Come with me,' says the woman slowly, 'come with me,'

I don't move, but I can just hear myself say *the virus...the virus...the virus* over and over again. Everyone will be dead in a couple of hours because of me.

'There's no virus dear, come with me...'

TWO POEMS

Nazik al-Malaika

(من الشمال الى اليمين) - الصف الامامي : شوقي ابي شقرا ، محمد
الماغوط ، يوسف الخال ، فؤاد رفقه ، ادونيس، فدوى طوقان،
لور غريب - الصف الخلفي : جورج صيدح ، نازك الملائكة ،

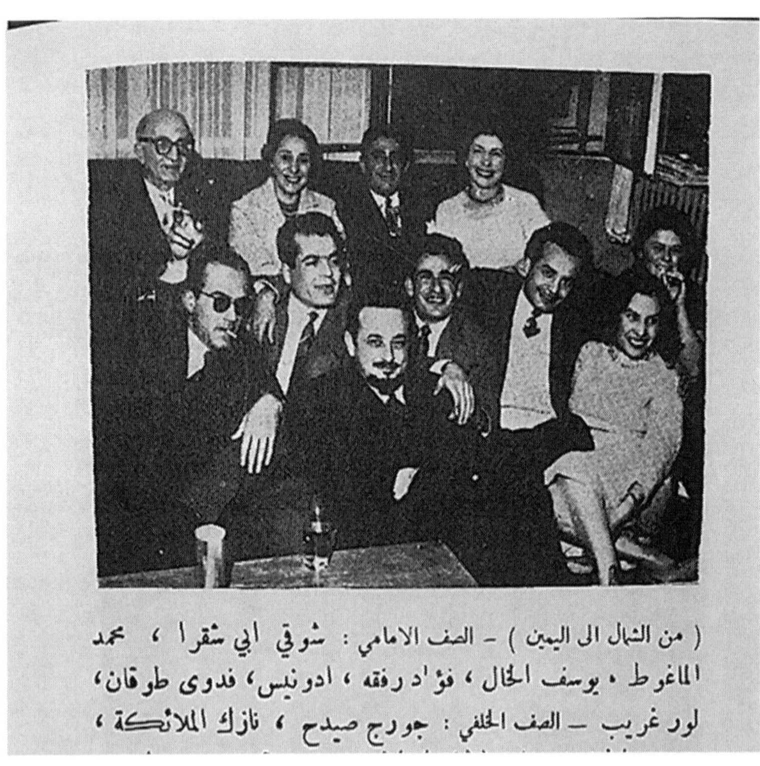

A gathering of Arab poets for a session of Beirut-based poetry journal Shiʿr's Thursday reading series in January 1960. Includes Yusif al-Khal, Adonis, Fadwa Tuqan, Nazik al-Mala'ika and Salma Khadra Jayussi

Revolt Against the Sun

A gift to the rebels

She stood before the sun, screaming out loud:
Oh Sun, my rebel's heart is just like you:
while young, it washed away much of my life,
its lights quenched the stars' thirst, ever renewed.
Careful – don't let the sadness in my eyes
or these copious tears deceive your sight.
This sadness is the form of my revolt,
to which the gods bear witness every night.

Careful, don't be deceived by my pale skin,
these quivering emotions, this dark frown.
If you see indecision, or the lines
of fierce poetic sadness on my brow,
know that it's feeling causing my soul's grief
and tears at life's terror – it's prophecy
that failed to fly, but stood up to resist
a life of sadness and melancholy.

My lips are fastened shut over their pain,
my eyes are thirsty for sweet drops of dew,
the evening left its shadow on my brow
and morning's killed off all my pleas to you.
I came to pour out my uncertainty
in nature, amid fragrances and shade,
but you, Sun, mocked my sadness and my tears
and laughed, from up above, at all my pain.

Even you, Sun? Alas, what misery!
You were the one I yearned for in my dreams,
you were the one whose name I once revered,
singing the praises of your smiling beams.
You were the one I once held sacred and
idolized as a refuge from all pain.

But now, crusher of dreams, melancholy,
darkness, and shadows are all that remain.

I will shatter the idol that I built
to you out of my love for radiance
and turn my eyes away from your bright light –
you're nothing but a ghost, splendor's pretense.
I'll build a heaven out of hidden hopes
And live without your luminosity.
We dreamers know we hold within our souls
divine secrets, a lost eternity.

Do not spread out your beams over my grove,
You rise for other than my poet's heart.
Your light no longer stirs feelings in me,
the night stars now inspire all my art.
They are the friends who guard me in the dark,
they understand the feelings that ignite
my spirit, they extend thin, silver threads
to guide my eyes through the enchanted night.

Night is life's melody, its poetry,
here gods of beauty roam to their content,
here uninhibited souls fly about
and spirits hover in the firmament.
How often I have wandered to forget
life's gloomy sorrows in the evening's dark,
upon my lips, a divine melody
recited by a caravan of stars.

How often I have watched stars as they pass
letting the twilight tune my incantations,
and watched the moon bidding the night goodbye,
and roamed the valleys of imagination.
The silence sends a shiver through my spine
beneath the evening's dome, so still and dark,

light dances, painting on my eyelids with
the dreamy palette of a peaceful heart.

And as for you, oh Sun… what can I say?
What can my feelings hope to find in you?
Don't be surprised that I'm in love with night,
goddess of cruel flames that melt us through.
You rend our dreams on the horizon line,
you decimate what we build in the dark,
you shatter magic visions, ghostly dreams,
and break the silence in a poet's heart.

All of your dancing lights look pale, oh Sun,
compared to my resistance and its fire.
Your mad flames can't tear up my melody
so long as my hands grasp this singing lyre.
And when you flood the earth, remember this:
My temple has no room for your cruel light
I aim to bury the past you revealed
And live beneath the canopy of night.

(8 July 1946)

Cholera

in the night
listen to echoed moans as they fall
in the depths of the dark, in the still, on the dead
voices rise, voices clash
sadness flows, catches fire
echoed cries, stuttered cries
every heart boils with heat
silent hut wracked with sobs
spirits scream through the dark everywhere
voices weep everywhere

this is what death has done
they are dead, they are dead, they are dead
let the strained Nile lament over what death has done

in the dawn
listen to passing feet as they fall
in the still of the dawn, watch and hear the procession of tears
ten are dead, twenty dead
countless dead, hear the tears
hear the pitiful child
they are dead, many lost
they are dead, there is no future left
bodies strewn everywhere, everywhere the bereaved
not a moment to mourn, not a pause
this is death's handiwork
they are dead, they are dead, they are dead,
all humanity suffers the crimes death commits

cholera
lies with corpses in terrible caves
death becomes medicine for eternity's hush
cholera lies awake
unavenged, overflowing with hate
pouring over the Delta's sweet soil
crying out, agitated, insane
it is deaf to the voices that mourn
as its talons leave scars everywhere
in the poor peasant's shack, in the landowner's house
nothing but cries of death, pouring out,
they are dead, they are dead, they are dead
as death takes its revenge wearing cholera's face

silence, still
nothing left but the trace of *Allahu akbar*
as the gravedigger too lies in eternal sleep
there is no one to help

the muezzin is dead
who will eulogize them?
nothing left now but shuddering sobs
the poor child has no mother, no dad
and tomorrow disease will no doubt snatch him too

evil cholera, what have you done?
you've left nothing in Egypt but sadness and death
they are dead, they are dead, they are dead
this is what death has done, and my heart is in shreds

(1947)

Extract from *Revolt Against the Sun: The Selected Poetry fo Nizik al-Malaika: A Bilingual Reader*, edited by Emily Drumsta, Saqi Books, London, 2020

CELTICS, SAINTS AND SUFIS

Carol Rumens

Ghazal: The Reluctant Anchorite

That old, corrupt pleasure – don't you remember – to show yourself!
The clothes curtseyed: *we'll help you conceal and show yourself.*

With make-up like precious oil in the lamp of Best Lights
You were calm as brocade. Like a queen, you'd bestow yourself.

Not one of the notable planets – Venus, Mars, Jupiter – or
His retinue of moons – no – but you surely owe yourself

A whiff of ineffable you-ness, which others sense
On the air: it's not the same when you video yourself.

The looking-glass hazes with glitterless star-dust. Perhaps
You're a mould in a bathroom crack, learning to grow yourself,

Or, like some darting rodent the cats and time forgot,
You're the tiny museum where you hastily stowed yourself?

'Oh, brave new normal!' chorus the screen-walled pundits,
The digital demons of Lockdown. 'Log in, and follow yourself!

Zoom till you drop. Shop will you swoon. Buy the moon
Without moving.' I find a puddle in which to throw myself.

'If you were a dervish', the sage says, 'would you stop
Before you'd touched every god, above, alongside, below yourself?'

His hand's on my shoulder. I'm free to choose silence, or sing
The gifts that name Allah: they name the things you owe yourself –

Forgiveness, protection, wisdom. Or why not become a Welsh saint,
Buarth Gwarchau the island to which you row yourself!

But first there's this form to fill in online, dry desert-father penance
Requiring your age, ethnicity, gender. Hallo, Yourself!

On Touch-Write, your fingernail glides a black lipstick! Amazed,
You comb out the curl of your name, and more or less know yourself.

(Note: *Buarth Gwarchau* – Welsh meaning 'shelter for cows,' the name of my cottage)

Cwyddau: The Happy Hermit

Isn't it virtue to sing
  With cormorant and herring

Lithe divers, flashing fishes?
  What saint needs a diocese?

Priests throw us a frayed lifeline:
  Be re-born! Be washed divine!

Oh, miracles, oh, stories!
  Catch hold of none but the sea's.

I tore the tongue from my head
  (A hermit-crab translated).

In the rock-pools, *morlo d'wi;*
  My mouth drips, my breath's fishy.
There are no cries of 'Repent!'

Across the packed escarpment

But shrieked arrival, scolding
Theatres of blue-black wing.

I work with smaller devils,
Pierce them, scourge the bright scales

With my hazel-stick: gasped death
Is their Bedydd Sanctiadd.

(*Notes: Cwyddau* – Welsh poetic form, 7 syllables per line, couplets rhyming an accented and unaccented word. *Morlo d'wi* – I am a seal. *Bedydd Sanctiadd* – Holy Baptism)

Hafiz, to Rumi

(*'God has given us a darker wine so potent that, / Drinking it, we leave the 2 worlds* '- *Mathnawi* IV, 2683–96, *The Essential Rumi*, tr. Coleman Barks)

I'm not looking, Mawlawi, for sanctity in this jar,
not thirsting for Light, for dark-browed, dimpled Laylah,

Or Death, or Yesterday. No crimson summer rose
transforms my good brown cup. Sniff it! The vintners propose

this year's Shiraz (like last year's) an exceptional vintage.
So when, cup drained, I act the little tin sage –

though you wish there were more ghazals in Paradise –
don't strain your ears for my profundities!

I'll stick with our Sufi dress-code: metaphors
should be simple wool, not silk. I remember one of yours…

The day's long transport done, at last untied,
the camel smiles at whatever the sands provide.

It pokes around, kneels down, laps up the divine
saltiness of the desert thorns, the same as I sip wine.

Mawlawi, you told us to dance when we commemorate
your funeral every year: we call it 'The Wedding Night'.

Mix 'drinking' , 'praying' , 'death' and 'love': relent,
and yield to this camel, Hafiz, the winning argument.

('Drink the wine that moves you/ as a camel moves when it's been untied,/and is just ambling about'. *Mathnawi* IV, 2683-96, *The Essential Rumi,* tr. Coleman Barks)

Rabi'a, Disarmed

1.

She raised the torch, fingers and knuckles stung
by the sparks spat back from the roaring wood.
The jar that swayed on the palm of her other hand
tried to rip the tendons from her shoulder,
and almost tipped and smashed. She sang away the pain
and some of her sisters, keeping well back, joined in.

'How fierce young women are' From the inner room,
that voice was mocking her. It persisted gently,
'Why do you want to burn down the walled garden?
Why do you want to quench hell?' She stamped her numb foot.
'You know what I know, my lord! They're snakeskins, hiding you,
veils that cover the eyes and mouths which love you!'
'But what if the sweet shade nicknamed Paradise
is one of the faces I choose? What if hell is

one of the bodies – perhaps Rabi'a's body?
Rest your arms, put the fire out, take a breath;
hold your hand deep in the sooty water,
the cold, kind water which un-blisters skin.'

From the room where her lord whispered her language, smiles
flowed through Rabi'a like sweet mint tea.
Rest here,
he said, *where the quince-trees drink from the aquaduct.*
Let us both be naked.

2

'When people tell me they admire my poems
I bow politely, trying not to show
how little their opinion means to me.
There's only one whose praise I listen out for.

I know the voice in which he sometimes speaks
may be my own. I'm always distant, careful --
except when signing off a poem. Oh, then,
wild and sick as a bride whose groom is late,
I listen, listen, even for *that voice*.

But on the subject of my poems, even
that voice has no opinion whatsoever.'

REVIEWS

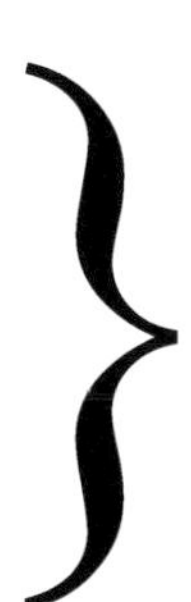

BRAIN FOG

Samia Rahman

It was at the Muslim Institute Winter Gathering on 12 December 2020, regrettably virtual by necessity but still wonderfully vibrant, that writer Medina Whiteman pondered the impact on the creative process of the interminable endlessness of lockdown. She was speaking as part of a panel exploring storytelling in the age of pandemia and described how distracted from her usual productivity she had become. Searching for the right words to capture the delirium of tedium that 2020 has turned out to be, she chanced upon the perfect metaphor for the prevailing impact of lockdown on prolificacy. 'It's like brain fog' she said, and almost every writer, creative and individual of an artistic disposition knew exactly what she meant.

In fact, this brain fog has been far from confined to a section of the global population that categorises itself according to any perceived imaginative ability. 2020 has been a year of unpredictability and unfathomable anxiety stretching out into every corner of the world. Extreme scenarios are being played out on every continent, often compounding already difficult circumstances as populations navigate the virus whilst in the midst of crisis brought on by poverty, conflict and disaster. The irony is not lost on me that there are many who are looking wearily at those of us jolted out of our first world bubbles. What is new to us is old to the oppressed and occupied. Life has slowed, become smaller, less tangible, and although there is no denying that for many this era has signalled a welcome pause from the frenetic pace of life, for others it has triggered psychological anguish, job insecurity and loneliness. If you've watched Groundhog Day, you might have felt replicated within that very premise, or perhaps stuck in the Netflix series (and who hasn't gorged on Netflix and other streaming channels this year) *Russian Doll*. We're living in an extended present which seems to be without any end in sight, with only a flicker of optimism that the promise of a vaccine offers, and obviously the vaccine is not a magic potion that will make all of this go away. Most, if not all of us, have had moments of feeling overwhelmed by this dystopian situation we find ourselves in. Those of us without caring responsibilities are sleeping more yet report feeling lethargic and fatigued. Concentration levels have faltered and for many 2020, well pretty much since March, has felt like one long blur, not unlike that period between Christmas and New Year when you don't quite know what day it is.

The dichotomy of seemingly incompatible emotions churning within us is difficult to comprehend but three novelists have done what I could hardly fathom to be possible and put into words at break-neck speed our collective global distress. It is perhaps not a coincidence that the short books, each containing a series of searing, thought-provoking compositions, should be written by women who are both storytellers and essayists. In their intimate and contemplative respective publications Arundhati Roy, Elif Shafak and Zadie Smith bring alive the mood of 2020 in all its ugliness and beauty. Sitting down to read *Intimations*, a collection of six essays written by Zadie Smith during the early phases of lockdown, I find it extraordinary that anyone could capture in words the utter bewilderment so many of us have attempted to articulate in response to the ongoing goings-on. Smith does so effortlessly yet with an eloquent hesitancy and introspection that bears witness to all that we struggle to make sense of. She allows her stream of consciousness to dart from seismic events, which, for brief moments make it seem as if things cannot be the same ever again, to the minutiae of individual lives that cascade into the deeply personal. We are introduced to everyday people of casual interactions with their coping mechanisms and concealed tragedies. We feel the gut-punch of the murder of George Floyd, yet another black man killed by US police who once again chose not to walk down the path of de-escalation. The anger and frustration that galvanised the Black Lives Matter movement spills out from the pages. And all this against a backdrop of the pandemic. Smith reflects on the elasticity of time, the quantifying of labour and the blurring of all work/life balance. Reading her soothing, consoling words helps the brain fog take shape in our minds. At last a long-awaited diagnosis after stumbling through a disorienting onslaught of indistinct symptoms.

This fog that doesn't seem to lift is given voice in these works of prose. Much has been spoken about a mental health crisis, not just as a result of Covid, but as a consequence of the violence of all that is 'normal' in our lives, such as institutional racism and inequality and the labelling of non-conformity as 'crazy'. All lay bare the limitations of the here and now in which we enact our existences. Perhaps this will herald the moment we finally learn we can exist outside our own perceptions of ourselves. So much of these existential disruptions are our own doing, but where life goals are yanked out of reach and improvised compromise takes the place of meticulously planned schemes, we would do well to grasp the opportunity to initiate new stories. Just as hell resides in the deepest recesses of our internal imagination, might our discomfort enable us to locate and trace the stories of the violent past in our disturbed present, while staring down the barrel into the most uncertain of futures. As Smith writes: 'the profound misapprehension of reality is what, more or less, constitutes the mental state we used to call "madness", and when the world itself turns unrecognisable, appears to go "mad". I find myself wondering what the effect is on those who never in the first place experienced a smooth relation between the phenomena of the world and their own minds.'

Arundhati Roy, *Azadi: Freedom. Fascism. Fiction*, Penguin, 2020
Elif Shafak, *How To Stay Sane In An Age of Division: The Powerful Pocket-sized Manifesto*, Wellcome Collection, London, 2020
Zadie Smith, *Intimations: Six Essays*, Penguin, 2020

Zadie Smith's quiet and contemplative untangling of the knots of where we find ourselves presents us with the glimpse of a possible future. The year 2020 was one in which everything that symbolised 'normal' was revealed to be truly limited and unable to withstand unforeseen or destabilising events. Yet this 'normal' is pretty much what we base our short term plans on, this assumption that things will carry on as they are, only to be blindsided when chaotic events, big or small, storms such as Covid-19, throw into chaos all the plans we've confidently carved out for ourselves. Our five-year plans, our career and life goals, everything we feel we are entitled to expect our futures to hold.

Now is the perfect opportunity to consider how we cultivated this concept of 'normal' that we are so desperate to get back to. The environmental journalist and author George Monbiot recently produced a short video examining the act of self-harm that is Brexit and the capitalist interests that fuelled the Leave campaign's victory. His scalpel-like analysis concluded with a question that keeps me awake at night: why is in-depth and contextual reporting absent from our major news channels?

I know the answer, but it doesn't make it any better. The digital age has contracted our attention spans as we gorge on a diet of bite-sized, oven-ready (mis)information. Arundhati Roy and Elif Shafak concern themselves with the dumbing down of our sources of information, and its horrific consequences that manifest as the 'normal' times of what was before. The title of Arundhati Roy's impassioned and blistering work is *Azadi*, the Urdu word for freedom. She details the rise and rise of Indian Prime Minister Narendra Modi and his sinister brand of Hindu fundamentalism. Roy tackles its consequences – populist authoritarianism, bigotry and parochialism – head-on in her exposition of India's occupation of Kashmir and the brutalising of its people, as well as targeting religious and ethnic minorities. In an age when facts and experts are swiftly dismissed as orchestrators of fake news, she addresses the way in which a novelist might approach the juxtaposition of the worlds that inhabit their imagination and the worlds that inhabit their reality, whatever they may be. She explains: 'I have never felt that my fiction and non-fiction were warring factions battling for suzerainty. They aren't the same, certainly, but trying to pin down the difference between them is actually harder than I imagined. Fact and fiction are not converse. One is not necessarily truer than the other, more factual than the other, or more real than the other. Or even, in my case, more widely read than the other. All I can say is that I feel the difference in my body when I'm writing.'

It's these limitations within our realities that we have truly come face to face with in the year of the virus. But instead of consigning it to the status of anomaly, a write-off, it should be one in which we finally accept the frailty, the unsustainability of our pre-Covid 'normal' and the ludicrousness of forcing a reinstatement of all that which is a mere continuation of what we had before. What a time to be alive, what potential for change. Yet, I fear we will be disappointed. When lockdown was first imposed there was a great deal of excitement at the way nature would reclaim the earth laid waste by human degradation. It wasn't to be and the climate crisis is as urgent as ever before. I suggested to my niece and nephew, who are nine and seven, that they keep a diary because in eighty odd years they will be the ones regaling future generations with stories of the infamous year 2020. Of course they didn't listen and prefer to document their experiences by playing Roblox, acting out pretend YouTube videos and other Gen Z activities that I am too archaic to appreciate. But really, as we get the sense that the chance to re-frame and remake 'normality' seems to be slipping through our fingers, all we have are our stories. And what Smith, Roy and Shafak achieve is the sharing of stories by making sure we can hear each other, interrogate the internal chatter of our ideas, and give each voice connection to the one we hear in our heads, the intimacy of familiarity, in what is the most strange and bewildering of times.

The prospect of a sudden and shocking collective convulsion, that could seemingly unite the world, whether it be dutifully observing lockdowns, reversing the climate crisis, or marching for black lives, was perhaps inconceivable before March 2020. Then, for a fleeting moment, everything that had bitterly divided us seemed to melt into irrelevance. After all, there was an unprecedented emergency on our doorstep that put so much into perspective. I happened to fly back to London from Berlin in early March, where I spent a long weekend contemplating exile with Arab friends crushed in spirit by the failures of the Arab Spring. Lockdown descended and I found much comfort in Twitter. By the end of the summer every crack that had been papered over by the so-called 'Blitz Spirit' was once more a gaping chasm. Although I still love all that is good about Twitter, social media maintains the potential to morph into a viper's nest of division and hate at the slightest provocation. In Elif Shafak's *How To Stay Sane In An Age of Division* the introspective balm of Zadie Smith's stunning wordplay becomes overtly political while Arundhati Roy's blend of magical realism, political non-fiction is deliciously characteristic of her work. That all three women are novelists is quickly evident in the mesmerising prose of their diverse narratives written during the recent long months of brain fog.

It is while reading Roy's compelling essays that I am taken back to George Monbiot's question. Surely if this type of critical thinking was a normalised part of our news consumption, the levels of ignorance that cause people to support the perpetrators of the structural injustices they endure, may be challenged. Since Modi came to power I have been refused a visa to visit India, the birthplace of my late father and all of my grandparents, ostensibly because my mother was born in Pakistan. Is this what my identity has been reduced to? Elif Shafak writes: 'A human being, every human being, is complicated – layers upon layers of ideas, feelings, perceptions, recollections, reactions, desires and dreams. By placing others into boxes we are denying them their own truths.' It is unquestionable that we are living in an age of bitter division, and although this is not a new phenomena, a wealth of factors unique to our contemporary era are exacerbating this explosion in right-wing, hate-fuelled populism. Despite the title of her book, Shafak doesn't offer any solutions to staying sane per se, but turns her attention to the entrenched and polarised nature of debate on social media as a wellspring of the problem. This is all a far cry from what was once hailed as social media's democratising promise.

Could it be that the virus will force us to confront our thirst for abstract connection without dialogue as we are, for the first time in our lives, deprived of real life person-to-person contact? Or perhaps it has further normalised non-human interaction as we retreat into our cyber-sanctuaries, shut the world of pandemia firmly out, resign ourselves to stagnating in a mire of uninformed, reactionary opinion, and surrender to the brain fog? As long as we have Roy, Shafak and Smith telling our stories, however, I have some optimism that the brain fog will eventually lift.

ELEMENTS OF CONVIVIALITY

Peter Coates

The Great Rethink by Colin Tudge is an absolute must for all those who are deeply concerned about humanity at large and the present state of the world. Whether humanity will be able to pull itself up by its own bootstraps is the thousand-dollar question. Colin Tudge, whilst recognising the enormity of the task ahead (including the necessary implications for the biosphere and the non-human fellow creatures on our planet) documents in this book a sentinel and clear sign of hope. A hope well-grounded and not a million miles from Rumi's assurance that 'ours is not a caravan of despair'.

It is a hope which involves a radical critique of the contemporary oligarchies of wealth and power. The modern politics of oligarchy premised as they often are on the awesome consumption and the demands of an exponential growth of the world population and, in turn, often (almost inevitably) exemplify a predominant mantra of the virtues of competition and perpetual economic expansion. All this is usually taken as the key to the ultimate survival and wellbeing of modernity itself.

In this connection it is interestingly noted in *The Great Rethink* that in 2020 the British medical journal *The Lancet* cited a report by 'the Norwegian Professor scientist Stein Emil Vollset of the University of Washington and his colleagues which predicted that human numbers will peak before the end of this century and then fall rapidly – in some countries by more than 50 per cent': the so called 'sigmoid' effect.

Colin Tudge, *The Great Rethink: A 21st Century Renaissance*, Pari Publishing, Pari, 2021

There is a kind of a holistic diagram in the book, with a host of sub-Venn diagrams, showing the interconnections and over-lapping areas of central concern to the success of the proposed *21st Century Renaissance.* Obviously, from even a precursory glance, the diagram implies the necessity of a high level of coordination and mutual understanding and a Great Conversation to take place to accompany the Great Rethink by means largely of the World-Wide-Web. And that means the breaking down of disciplinary barriers and barriers of all kinds. The outer encompassing circle of this intriguing diagram is labelled 'flourishing biosphere' to indicate unambiguously that what we are dealing with, at all levels, is a holistic living dynamic reality with at its centre the well-being and flourishing of all human life and all that makes human life possible. This leaves open the question of a metaphysics of the Sacred to which we will return.

At this point let us be quite clear: this is not (as some might take it to be) an unrealisable Utopianism. Rather it is an evolving prototype for the future. And for such an evolving prototype to be well-grounded and established the findings and recommendations of Ecology are, as we know, essential. Essential that is for the survival of the planet and ourselves and all else.

Let us consider some thoughts on the nature of what is termed the Ecological Crisis. In the section on climate change Tudge cites Greta Thunberg's memorable reprimand to the powers that be:

> People are suffering. People are dying and ecosystems are collapsing. We are in the beginning of a mass extinction and all you can talk about is the money and fairy tales of eternal economic growth.... How dare you look away and come here saying that you're doing enough when the politics and solutions needed are still nowhere in sight!

This is a reprimand that this book takes seriously. And to it I would like to add the following.

Let us notice that the idea of unity, and if you wish the acknowledgment of our common universal humanity, is increasingly brought to our attention in all kinds of twenty-first-century nooks and crannies. This point is well-recognised throughout the book. There is definitely emerging a sense and recognition of the interconnectedness and unity of life as a whole and of the indissoluble relationship between man and nature. We see images of fundamental unity emerging in the study of the very small and the very great – in cosmology, physics, biology, ecology, economics, in the global inter-dependence of diverse socially, culturally and geographically disparate communities and even in some ecumenical contexts. More generally, we see this in the breaking down of barriers of all kinds, including gender. There is a kind of healthy 'unity-in-diversity' and 'diversity-in-unity' replacing constricting dualisms. In many ways holistic understandings have become more prevalent. We need to recognise this tendency when considering the all-too-obvious divisions of the age in which we live. We may even suggest that the ecological crisis itself is, in some partial and potential sense, a unifier in so far as it is ultimately larger than the divisions which separate us: we cannot act alone and we are all affected. Some such embryonic degree of unity– a feeling for the oneness of Life in all its diversity and a recognition of our common humanity, is in many people, I suspect, part of a taken-for-granted common sense. Not much talked about perhaps but a powerful subterranean current – a potential antidote to intolerance and division. People can gather in the name of their common humanity in spite of their sometimes-intransigent ideological divisions: what has happened very recently in Northern Ireland is a promising example. Sometimes it takes great preparation for something seemingly solid 'to melt into air' and sometimes it happens in the twinkling of an eye, 'or even less' as it is sometimes tantalisingly expressed. I cannot think of a better description of how great shifts in human consciousness and ideas take place than this. If this point can be summarised it is that the ecological crisis acts itself as a mirror, or even a magnifying glass, for the necessity of a fundamental change in human consciousness and awareness. It is a crisis capable of bringing the human species to its senses: it is more than an ecological crisis – it is a mirror to the tawdry nature of much of our stewardship of the world. It is therefore a mirror to ourselves, to our state and to our attitudes.

This clearly supports an *agroecology* (which is of particular interest to our author) 'to treat all farms as ecosystems and as far as possible treat all agriculture as a positive contributor to the biosphere and to create landscapes that on the one hand provide crops and livestock that people want (which is the *agro* bit) but which are also as wildlife friendly and diverse as possible, and close to the putatively pristine (natural) state'. And the book advocates a wild-friendly economy.

It is no surprise that our author remarks that Ecology is the most profound biological advance of the twentieth and twenty-first century, revealing 'how all organisms on Earth mesh together and interact with their surroundings each individual with its own *niche* (my word)…but absolutely depended on the others, each part of a far larger whole.'

It is worth noting here that in his balanced reading of Darwin he reminds us that Darwin also stressed the importance of co-operation in nature. This becomes a central observation in countering the 'metadarwinian' claim (as he calls it) 'that all creatures including human beings must compete, compete, compete for earth's limited resources'. We can begin to see here the essential direction of travel: the true nature of human kind or the human species is to be construed as *conviviality.*

There are a number of very interesting sections devoted to elaborating its conceptual and practical significance: the biology of conviviality, sex and sociality, sociality and cooperation are the keys to Intelligence and the politics of conviviality. But these considerations rest on the kind of view of humankind, for example, in which, as Adam Smith (cited by Tudge) posits, there are 'those principles in his nature which interest him in the fortunes of others, and render their happiness necessary to him, though he derives nothing from it except the pleasure of seeing it'. And these 'principles' are essential to the full and proper functioning of humankind. They cannot be reduced to its more animal nature. This would be to commit a kind of mereological fallacy: the mistake of reducing the whole to one of its parts. And equally this is not to deny that animals can co-operate and care for each other. Although one may want to add that in our case our animal nature may become predominant and our more essential conviviality remain largely unawakened. This is why, in part, Socrates arguably insisted that the unexamined life is not worth living although I don't think he mentions the exact term conviviality. But celebration is certainly part of the human conviviality of the Socratic/Platonic universe: consider their feasts and libations and Diotimas' riveting convivial and celebratory conversations on beauty in the *Symposium*. So generally, although perhaps the term *conviviality* may seem a little unusual it is particularly apt as it embraces both the social nature of being human and elevated states of consciousness including the enjoyment in witnessing the happiness of others.

There is so much more in this book of considerable and informative interest but to make this review manageable I propose to concentrate selectively on Part V: Mindset sections 12, 13 and 14 which covers morality, science and metaphysics. It is in Part V that we approach the nub of the matter that is the necessity to bring all this together into a coherent unifying metaphysical vision subject to ongoing revision in the light of future developments and he takes his redefinition of the traditional descriptor Perennial Wisdom to mean a perpetual, never-ending open quest, for-ever work-in-progress which avoids any form of authoritative dogmatism. A dogmatism which he sees, of course, as an obvious limitation of historical religion. But I don't think Tudge talks in the same vein about what he calls a 'Sense of the Sacred'. He is, for example, in total agreement with Seyyed Hossein Nasr's penetrating insight that 'metaphysics as an independent discipline has largely gone missing; and this he suggests, is the greatest single cause of the disastrous state in which the world now finds itself'. And it is *metaphysics* not dogma which interests Tudge and many others I suspect. But Nasr raises another point concerning the cause of this disaster that is 'the disappearance of *gnosis* from the mainstream of Western thought' and which I myself suggest , on its noticeable resurgence in the West, largely through the stimulus of the writings of Ibn 'Arabi and Rumi, may shed an entirely different light on the possibility of a universal metaphysics beyond dogma. And it is a metaphysics whose fundamental ethics revolves round self-realisation: we have to become what we already are. Both these seminal figures are mentioned in the *The Great Rethink* and by Nasr himself. We shall come back to this idea of a universal metaphysics after we have looked a bit more closely at what the book has to say about morality and then about the nature and limitations of science.

Tudge turns, but not uncritically, in this section to Jeremy Bentham's arithmetic of human happiness: the famous principle of 'the greatest happiness of the greatest number'. Tudge himself favours Virtue Ethics and the centrality of Compassion. For Bentham, however, if you want to know what ethical act you should follow (or ought to bring about) it should be that act or acts which lead to the greatest happiness of the greatest number. And, if you happen to assume that generally what makes citizens happy is an increase in their personal wealth (not an uncommon assumption) then this can deeply affect government policy-making and in essence allow some kind of loose arithmetic verification. However, It may have been useful here also to cite John Stuart Mill's *On Liberty* in which he famously and influentially introduces the whole question of the *quality* and variety of human happiness, not simply its arithmetical value. And in so doing accords a healthy liberty to 'experiments in living'. Experiments which may run counter to the conventional wisdom of the times. And as it is sometimes starkly expressed 'better to be a Socrates dissatisfied than a pig satisfied'. Mill, of course, attempts to provide a utilitarian principle for deciding which form of happiness has the qualitatively higher value.

But to bring this round to the concerns of the book we can see that the setting up (by Colin Tudge and his wife Ruth) of the College for Real Farming and the Oxford Real Farming Conference (ORFC) could well be seen as constituting 'an experiment in living': to be judged perhaps by the passage of time? Or better still, to be judged by the more-than-humanist maxim (close to the heart of William James) – that 'we shall know them by their fruits'.

Next we need to move on to what I said about science and importantly the philosophy of science which our author considers inseparable for arriving at a balanced view of science. I will not dwell on the treatment of Logical Positivism for the simple reason that it is considered moribund these days and its attempt to eliminate metaphysics from the philosophical agenda is hardly persuasive and itself unverifiable. But there is a development in more recent philosophy of science which avoids the danger of scientism and which presents us with an understanding of the dispositional nature of reality as a whole and which casts an interesting and fruitful light on any metaphysics of unity. As Rom Harré (1927–2019), British philosopher and psychologist, who taught philosophy of science at Oxford University, points out 'post-Newtonian quantum physicists can no longer seek for "things" but must look for dispositions and affordances and that … we have more reason for thinking that the universe is composed of a field of energy rather than thinking of it as composed of lots of chunky bits of matter' and he concludes that the world is a very rich source of dispositions, but in physics 'it makes no sense to ask what it is really beyond the affordances; this we cannot say it remains an insoluble mystery'. If we generalise a little and conceive of reality outside the universe of physics to be also dispositionally multifaceted and capable of revealing different aspects of itself, depending on the way it is approached, as it is with our encounter with ourselves and others and with music, art, literature, philosophy, religion, and mathematics the possibilities are literally endless. But the truth is that it soon becomes apparent that some approaches may reveal more of realities' deeper dispositional riches than others and even reveal apparently contradictory aspects.

To return to the book's discussion on metaphysics, we can usefully turn to Ibn 'Arabi's metaphysics of unity as being a dispositional view of the whole of created existence. God says 'I was a hidden treasure and I wanted to be known and so created the world that I might be known': so the whole of existence has value and purpose. It is a theophanic disposition 'to appear as'. It is a seamless metaphysics of Beauty which rests upon the reality that there is only 'One, Unique, Absolute, Infinite Existence'. The hallmark of such an extraordinary elevated viewpoint requires that Transcendence when asserted by the human intellect must always be accompanied by Immanence. As Rumi puts it, the two worlds are One. The essential status of Man is as a bridge or isthmus between Heaven and earth – paradoxically He and not-He.

Generally, with regard to the status of metaphysics Tudge suggests that 'many feel at one with the core ideas of metaphysics (the sense of transcendence, oneness, and ultimate mystery) and yet reject the particular doctrines of any one religion. This might be because some people have a strong distaste for dogma but it certainly would not be expressed in this reductively truncated way by Ibn 'Arabi. His universalism includes all religions (and the reason for their diversity) and is not tied to external or figurative belief and is not limited to historical religion or even to the kaleidoscope of personal belief. Ibn Arabi's metaphysics emphasises their root embodiment, ground and source and their fundamental mystery and primordiality. It embraces all reality at whatever level. And because of this 'the gnostic cannot stay tied to any one form of belief' lest a great good escapes him or her. In fact, Tudge himself includes in his book what are perhaps the most widely quoted lines from the *Tarjuman al-Ashwaq* (The Interpreter of Ardent Desire) of Ibn 'Arabi:

> My heart is a pasture for gazelles and a convent for Christian monks; a temple for idols and the pilgrim's Ka'aba, the tablets of the Torah and the book of the Qur'an. I follow the religion of Love. Whatever way Love's camels take that is my religion and my faith.

For Ibn 'Arabi, Self-knowledge is the central key in our possession which enables us epistemic access to, what is known traditionally, as the Unity of Existence or Being. But what is received depends crucially on the aptitude and receptivity of the receiver: the colour of the water takes on the colour of the receptacle as the great ninth century Persian Sufi, Junayd of Baghdad, said: 'to express the matter in a different way, there is no path to knowledge of God but knowledge of self … for He made yourself signify your knowledge of Him'. This is an extremely interesting and far reaching metaphysical principle.

Bearing in mind Colin Tudge's understanding of the meaning of Perennial Wisdom and having taken him at his word 'that the ideas of metaphysics and more specifically religion must be taken very seriously and acted upon' let us just bring things together. Well there is much I have not commented upon given the necessary economy of a review. But there is a wealth of detail in this book. It is well-structured and well-written and well-informed and exhibits a lightness of touch, and a seriousness of intent. This book ought to be required reading and as we carefully note: 'the intention is not to lay down the law and to tell everyone what to think for that would be hugely presumptuous, but to suggest an agenda and action for others to improve upon'. Nevertheless, the book is about human potential and human flourishing and aims to let us see for ourselves what the score is. And when a larger metaphysical landscape like Ibn 'Arabi's is brought into the picture then as Plotinus astutely remarks: the vision is there for those who will see it.

WHITE MUSLIMS

Josef Linnhoff

Islam is a universal faith that does not see race. 'Praise be to God, Lord of the worlds', the Qur'an declares in its opening verse. Not Lord of the Quraysh, Arabs or indeed any group that seeks to tribalise the divine. The Prophet stressed racial equality among believers. Notions of superiority through race or lineage are the real idols that Islam came to destroy. But against this stands the reality of our racialised world. For several centuries, whiteness has been attributed with culture, civilisation, beauty and reason. At its extreme, this has underpinned genocides, a slave trade, apartheid and a so-called civilising mission in which most of the Muslim world fell under European imperial rule. The latter was termed the 'white man's burden'. Islam may not see race – but Muslims do.

Medina Tenour Whiteman's *The Invisible Muslim: Journeys Through Whiteness and Islam*, explores what is means to be a white Muslim. Whiteman's interest stems from her experiences as the daughter of Anglo-American Sufi converts, born in Granada and raised in a 'whiter-than-white' area of Essex. She tells of struggling to find a sense of identity, never feeling at home in either Western or Muslim cultures. The book expresses this by the term 'invisible Muslim' and by a recurring motif of veils. Not the headscarf, but the figurative veils used to separate Us from Them. Veils of race, class and privilege separate Whiteman from Muslims of colour. The veil of religion separates her from other whites:

> There is a veil that recurs throughout my life…When I am among white people, I've seen on so many occasions this veil dropping when the penny drops. Faces change subtly, or not so subtly. Fingers start nervously fidgeting. All kinds of thoughts and questions being visibly running through the interlocutor's face: Are they a *progressive* Muslim?

Part memoir and part travelogue, the book traces Whiteman's life-long search for belonging via her travels across the Muslim world, to Bosnia,

Tibet, Tanzania and southern Spain, among other places. Chapters mix autobiography with history, social commentary and occasional Sufi wisdom. Throughout, Whiteman brings sharp insight, empathy and a serious intellect. She is also a beautiful writer. So how does whiteness shape one's experiences as a Muslim? How can white Muslims face the legacy of racial injustice and forge bonds with Muslims of colour? In what way does Islam act as a bridge to followers of different racial backgrounds? The book probes all these questions. Much of the discussion touches on broader themes of race, religion, identity and belonging in the modern world. The focus is on how these relate to Muslims.

The Invisible Muslim comes at an important cultural moment. Global protests condemn the police killings of black civilians in the US. Notions of 'white privilege' and 'systemic racism' have moved from academic and activist circles to the mainstream. Colonial history is under the spotlight as never before. Islam is rarely invoked in these debates but, as a racialised and subaltern community, much of this is relevant to Muslims. Throughout the book Whiteman grapples with her white heritage:

> I started to feel disgusted at my ethnicity, at the atrocities perpetrated by white people.

> Some years back I even did a DNA test, hoping I would find something that might break the monotony of my Anglo-American whiteness – something I would want to honour.

> I have often wished that I could escape the badge of whiteness that I carry on my face. How can I take pride in my Anglo-American roots? Not only have innumerable injustices been wreaked in the name of my ethnicity, but…I am directly descended from people who materially benefited from slavery.

But the book is about more than white guilt. Opening chapters explore how whiteness operates within Muslim spaces. We learn of how reactions to white Muslims in wider Muslim circles range from fetishisation to denial. On the one hand, the book gives a vivid account of white Muslim privilege: white Muslims can evoke a special celebration from Muslims of colour and are often held as prized assets in the community. Friendship requests and marriage proposals are common. White converts are a tiny percentage of the community but among its most famous names. The upshot of this is the treatment extended to other groups. As Whiteman notes, non-white converts receive far less attention and anti-black racism remains common in Asian and Arab circles. Yet this is not the whole story. On the other hand, the book also addresses the common view that whiteness somehow invalidates Islam, that whites are too much of a novelty to be 'real' Muslims. We read of white Muslims being interrogated upon entering mosques, shunned during religious festivals and facing suspicions of spying on the community. In Whiteman's case, they are also called 'half-Muslim'. Neither response, of course, offers a real sense of belonging and Whiteman speaks eloquently of her struggle for a space to be her true, authentic self. This also holds up a mirror to the wider Muslim community. Celebrating whiteness seems a sad reflection of how some Muslims of colour view themselves. Denial or exclusion points to a narrow, racialised conception of the faith.

Medina Tenour Whiteman, *The Invisible Muslim: Journeys Through Whiteness and Islam*, Hurst, London, 2020

White Muslims challenge the stereotype of a racialised, immigrant Islam. For this reason the book also looks at their reception in mainstream society. Here the tensions continue. 'Invisible' Muslims can of course pass off as non-Muslim but not all white Muslims are invisible. Some don visible markers of Islam like the *hijab*. A growing body of scholarship points to their facing a unique set of prejudices. British academic Leon Moosavi, for example, argues that white Muslims undergo a process of 're-racialisation' in wider society, losing part of their whiteness by identifying with a perceived foreign and non-white religion. Turkish scholar Esra Ozyurek notes that white Muslims are often accused of being 'traitors'. Ozyurek cites one ethnic German Muslim:

> I feel that as German Muslims we are doubly marginalised. First Germans push us aside, then Turks and Arabs turn their backs on us. That makes one feel very lonely. No one thinks about us when people talk about Muslims in Germany. We are totally invisible. Germans most often think we are crazy ... They call us traitors, people who left their culture behind and took someone else's.

The question arises: do white Muslims remain 'white' as such and retain their access to privilege? Terms like 'white trash' or 'chav' already point to a layered conception of whiteness – could 'white Muslim' be a similar category? The book notes this point but argues against it. White Muslims are 'tainted' by the association with Islam, Whiteman concedes, but they still enjoy privilege. Their whiteness means they are not stopped and searched, less likely to be victims of anti-Muslim attacks and avoid the structural barriers faced by ethnic minorities. But perhaps there is no real disagreement here, only a difference in emphasis. That is, Whiteman stresses the white Muslim retention of privilege while others point to the relative status-deficit that associating with Islam entails. The lesson is that some whites are 'more white' than others.

The book captures many of the nuances of white Muslim identity. If there is something missing, however, it is a deeper treatment of the topic of conversion. More precisely, the real challenges or costs of converting to Islam. In the UK at least, most white Muslims will be converts and most converts will be white. And conversion is not easy. Converts embrace a new way of life, learn new ritual practices and join a stigmatised community. Above all, they risk the hostility of closest friends and family. Such stories are depressingly common. One hears of daughters evicted from the family home and sons performing their prayers in the dead of night, fearing the ire of the family. Tied to this is how the wider Muslim community often fails converts - beyond hugs and smiles, structures in place to guide, support and educate those new to the faith are rare. The book touches on converts in several places but the real challenge of conversion is not explored in any detail. The point is that many pay a high price for converting to Islam and many such converts will be white. One could argue their story is not just one of privilege. It also involves pain, sacrifice and the rejection of loved ones. Exploring this further makes for a richer discussion.

Related to this is the role converts play in replenishing and indigenising a faith. Islam did not become a global religion through Arabs. For only through conversion does a faith go global. Only when local Indonesians, Uzbeks and Senegalese adopt Islam and make it their own do these lands join the House of Islam. One senses a tension in the book on this point. Whiteman notes the role of converts in spreading the faith. She lauds how ethnic Arabs comprised a tiny minority of Muslim Spain and notes the tradition of British converts to Islam, a tradition that includes such luminaries as Abdullah Quilliam and Marmaduke Pickthall.

> Having a history of white converts might support the nascent identity of white Muslims today, proving proof – like the Spanish Muslims of Al-Andalus – that Islam can be indigenised on European soil.

Elsewhere, however, the book warns against what it calls 'white exceptionalism' or 'whitewashing Islam'. Consider the following:

> Particularly grating is the insinuation that we legitimise Islam to non-Muslims, that our whiteness makes Islam more palatable and less alien. Often white Muslims are asked to do dawah, or outreach, at the mosque, the underlying assumption that a white face is somehow more approachable...Here again white privilege rears its head – but with a special Islamic twist.

We should avoid the idea that Islam is ok *because* white people can be Muslim. This indulges white privilege and feeds into white supremacy. Yet the question is how to square the fear of 'whitewashing' Islam with the special role of converts. In a Britain that is 87% white, do whites have a unique role to play in naturalising Islam, or is this problematic? Is promoting white Muslims for dawah a case of white privilege, as claimed, or a way of changing perceptions and breaking barriers? Are white Europeans the Uzbeks and Senegalese of tomorrow, or is this a new form of colonising Islam, a 'white saviour' complex in Islamic guise? The book avoids giving clear answers. Readers can answer these questions for themselves.

Most chapters take the form of a travelogue documenting Whiteman's experiences of travelling, studying and living across the Muslim world, in Kenya and Tanzania, Tibet, Iran, Bosnia and southern Spain. These sites of Muslim 'marginalia' on the 'margins of the *ummah*', she writes, hold a special appeal. The central theme is one of exploring what Muslim identity means the world over as part of a deeper, personal search for belonging. For its indigenous European Islam, for example, Bosnia feels like a 'homecoming'. Finding a Muslim community in Ladakh in Indian-administered Kashmir also holds lessons:

> If Ladakhi Muslims build their mosques in a local style, write Arabic prayers on flags like Buddhists do, and live largely in the same way as do followers of a faith that seems so unlike Islam , then to be a British, Western or white Muslim is not such a new or heterodox notion. It is simply a matter of perspective.

In each locale Whiteman shares a faith with the locals but finds she is still separated by veils of class, race, language or culture. But the insights into Muslim 'marginalia' have a powerful effect: these chapters shatter the myth of a monolithic Islam. Discussions range from Sufism and slavery in East Africa, cosmetic surgery in Iran, ethnic cleansing in Bosnia, Spanish Muslim history to Muslim-Buddhist relations in Tibet. The image is one of Islam embedded across a rich range of languages, cultures and ethnicities. The effect is that white Muslims appear not so unique or special. In a global *ummah*, they are one small part of a much richer mosaic.

The issue for many today is not Islam as a global faith but whether Islam can ever be at home in the West. In Britain the 'Muslim question' has become the great question of our time. It is tied to other questions around immigration, multiculturalism, free speech, dress and sexuality. It has sparked a national debate about 'British values'. For this reason the book's final chapters examine Muslim identity in Britain. Here, too, Whiteman makes a valuable contribution. She argues 'something extraordinary' is happening, with British Muslims increasingly assertive, vocal and mobile. She points to their shaping public life in fields from politics (Sadiq Khan) to television (Nadiya Hussein), literature (Kamila Shamsie) to sport (Mo Farah). Cambridge boasts an eco-mosque. The art scene is flourishing with pioneers like Amber Khokhar designing works for Buckingham Palace. Spaces like the Inclusive Mosque Initiative and Rumi's Cave cater to different kinds of religious expression. For many in Britain, Islam retains the stigma of foreignness. To this, Whiteman has an eloquent response.

> The UK might not be the genetic parent of most British Muslims, but it has been a wet nurse, one that often feels more familiar than an absent parent who isn't always easy to communicate with.

Social customs and expectations are also evolving. We read that divorce rates are rising, marriage and career expectations are changing, dating apps abound and pre-marital sex is not as rare as one might think. One wonders: if this is what it meant by Muslim 'integration' in Britain, it would appear a *fait accompli*. But obstacles remain. The book discusses the problem of Islamophobia, citing data to show Muslims were victims of 47 per cent of hate crimes in 2019 while only 5 per cent of the population. A brief reference to 'conservative currents' perhaps understates the patriarchy, sectarianism and intellectual dryness that plague many Muslim spaces – what *Critical Muslim*'s Leyla Jagiella calls the 'wahhabitus'. One could add that places like Rumi's Cave represent still the margins, not the mainstream, of British Islam. Still, the book makes a strong case that we are witnessing a process of dynamic change in what it means to be a British Muslim. This process defies simple binaries or stereotypes. It is more complex and layered than what is found in a headline or government report. Again, white Muslims – just 8 per cent of the UK Muslim community – are only one small part of a wider story.

It is worth adding here that Britain too finds itself at a crossroads. Grappling with a post-Brexit future and an imperial past, demographic change, regional divisions, huge economic and cultural divides and the effects of Covid – what Britain means or stands for is far from clear. This may be good news for British Muslims. A country with a firm and fixed idea of itself (think French *laicite*) presents its own challenges. Or, it may be that an uncertain and divided Britain continues to seek Others on whom its many problems can be blamed. No one can predict where this will lead. But if British Muslims are in a state of evolution, as the book makes clear, so too is Britain itself. How the two interact will shape the future of the British Muslim experience.

The Invisible Muslim speaks to various audiences. Whiteman offers a moving account of her life-long search for belonging and there are lessons here for all those navigating multiple identities, particularly diasporic communities, those of mixed-heritage or third culture kids. More specifically, one hopes the book inspires a wider conversation about white Muslim identity. Many books on Islam are written *by* white Muslims. None, until now, have so directly tackled the complex area of whiteness and Islam. If there is to emerge an authentic white Muslim selfhood, neither 're-racialised' nor privileged, rooted in the West but sustained by a wider *ummah*, this book has a role to play. White readers in general will benefit from the clarion call to break the taboo around discussing race, to disrupt the myth that white is normative. If the purpose of writing is not just to entertain but to educate, to provoke and to share feelings and experiences, Whiteman has roundly succeeded. I have read many books since the start of lockdown. Few have stirred as much questioning, introspection and enjoyment as this.

POWERFUL IDOLS

Sara Mohr

To the casual browser, *The Idols of ISIS* first appears to be a difficult read about the titular notorious Islamic extremist group. However, despite the title, Aaron Tugendhaft dedicates this monograph not to ISIS, but to a thorough discussion of images, weaving a story about the power of political images, including their destruction and manipulation, in a tale that truly brings Assyria to the internet. *The Idols of ISIS* comes to us at a timely moment, as scholars are sounding the alarm about how the internet delivers certain images to our lives, and as the scholarly and museum worlds begin to reckon more fully with their colonial pasts. As a historian of ancient Iraq, I found myself enamoured with the contrasts and comparisons Tugendhaft so expertly draws between the Iraq that ISIS wants you to see and the ancient Iraq that the world is so eager to claim as its own glorious past.

The prologue opens with a fitting anecdote. We find Tugendhaft at a lecture by the Iraqi art historian, Zainab Bahrani, at the Institute for the Study of the Ancient World at New York University. It is during this lecture that Tugendhaft becomes aware for the first time of the video of ISIS militants destroying ancient Assyrian statuary in Iraq's Mosul Museum. To highlight this moment is appropriate considering Bahrani's scholarly background in bringing attention to the stark contrast between the still-standing images of the ancient world and the symbols of modern conflict. She ends her omnibus work *Art of Mesopotamia* with the striking photo of an American helicopter hovering over the ziggurat of Babylon. In invoking Bahrani in his introduction, Tugendhaft sets us up for a fascinating and compelling comparison between ancient and modern destruction.

The destruction of specific imagery and statues is a particular kind of violence, and advertising it through video makes the violence that much more painful and present for many. Tugendhaft is quick to point out that the ISIS video serves as a kind of meta moment, showing how the militants wielding hammers are more like those whom they aim to destroy than they realise. In a relief from Sargon II's (722–705 BCE) palace at Khorsabad in northern Iraq, Tugendhaftt shows us another relief of three Assyrian soldiers smashing the sculpture of an enemy king. The question he poses is: why advertise this destruction? Just as ISIS does with their video of destruction, the Assyrian King Sargon II is using images to affect political feelings for those who see it: fear for those opposed, renewed enthusiasm from those who support. In these two images, separated by more than 2,500 years, Tugendhaft shows us that not only is there inherent power in the images we display, but also that in ISIS's decision to film the destruction of the Mosul Museum, they continue along the same thread of behaviour that connects them more deeply to the same reliefs they destroy.

Aaron Tugendhaft, *The Idols of ISIS: From Assyria to the Internet*, University of Chicago Press, 2020.

Bridging the gap further between Assyria and ISIS, Tugendhaft invokes Qur'anic stories and other Islamic doctrine. Complicating the issue in an interesting way, he notes that in the story of Ibrahim encountering idols, the text uses the terms 'image' and 'idol' interchangeably. Because Arabic and Akkadian, the ancient language of Assyria, share roots as east Semitic languages, it comes as no surprise that we have a similar linguistic relationship in Akkadian. The word *ṣalmu* is most simply translated as 'image.' However, the term encompasses so much more than just this single word. According to modern scholars of ancient Iraq, such as Zainab Bahrani, when *ṣalmu* is invoked, it refers to not just a representation of a person or thing, but something akin to a clone. The *ṣalmu* holds the essence of the person or thing it duplicates to the point that destroying it is the same as destroying the actual living thing it aims to represent. It is from this idea that we find ancient fears of image destruction.

As Tugendhaft points out, to destroy an image in Assyria was to drain it of its *melammu*, the life-giving, awe-inspiring radiance attributed to gods, kings, and their representations. Like *ṣalmu*, *melammu* is an intangible concept that evades modern translation. Tugendhaft describes it as 'an awe-inspiring radiance that emanated from kings and permeated the symbols of their royal power' . However, *melammu* extends beyond the realm of royalty and is much more closely associated with divinity. It more broadly refers to a kind of divine radiance or splendour. The use of this term is documented in cuneiform sources for thousands of years, showing a staggering continuity throughout Mesopotamian history. The *melammu* from a statue of a king or divine being gave that representation the sense of life implied by the term *ṣalmu*. As Tugendhaft describes the destruction at the hands of ISIS, you can imagine the sense of life and radiance with which the Assyrians imbued their images draining from their figures as hammers descended upon them. There is certainly a strong connection to be drawn between the destruction of cultural heritage and the loss of *melammu* that the Assyrians valued so strongly.

What remains after a statue is destroyed? The *melammu* has been lost and the figure is no longer a *ṣalmu*, but rather a collection of untethered stone pieces. When those pieces then appear in an internet video, Tugendhaft likens them to images drained of their *melammu* and reduced to data. This assertion then serves as a jumping off point for his discussion of just how prevalent data were in the ancient world. Largely, this book uses images in a masterful way that draws a single stream from ancient Mesopotamia to modern Iraq. However, this attempt to make a case for data in the ancient world falls flat as it stands next to the concepts of *ṣalmu* and *melammu*. Most striking among these attempts is the comparison between the vast array of mathematical texts from administrative contexts in Mesopotamia, and the algorithms that power Facebook. This comparison does a disservice to both the complexity of mathematical texts present in ancient Mesopotamia, and also distills the Facebook algorithm down to the bits and bytes that make up its AI. Just as Tugendhaft reminds us of images, there are people behind Facebook, creating and tweaking its algorithms in often problematic ways that affect how all of us think about the world.

The infamous video Tugendhaft uses as a base for this entire work, was brought to his attention through Facebook. He correctly notes that Facebook has been hailed as both a democratising force for political access and panned for its algorithms that distort our experience of the public realm. This distortion was probably no more on display than it was during the course of the 2016 US Presidential election, in which it used data and guidance from Cambridge Analytica to spread false information about both Hillary Clinton and Donald Trump. It comes as no surprise to see the same social media site invoked as a platform utilised by ISIS for the propagation of their own images. Equally fitting is Facebook's role as a battleground once again for another debate on the destruction of images: the controversy surrounding still-standing statues glorifying the Civil War, the fight over slavery, in the United States.

The debate about the role of US Confederate statues is perhaps one of the most polarising right now. Though only affording a brief discussion to this debate, *The Idols of ISIS* speaks deeply to this moment. The inclusion of such a similar modern discussion also touches upon the recent history of statue-toppling in Iraq. Readers of this work will likely be familiar with the image of a statue of Saddam Hussein falling and the story of the teamwork it required from both Iraqi citizens and American soldiers. As Tugendhaft points out, one aspect of this story stands out from all other examples: 'No one complained about the destruction of Iraqi cultural heritage'. It is points like these that really serve to pull the reader into the complexity that Tugendhaft sees in the interplay between ISIS, ancient Assyria, modern Iraqi history, and how it plays out on our screens. But how is it that we came to know this recent instance in Iraqi Images. Electronic images on social media and online newspaper publications. Once again, as Tugendhaft does so well throughout, the situation is further complicated. When we think of weapons used in the destruction of statuary, we think of hammers and rope. Rarely do we acknowledge the ways in which the digital forms of this destruction are weaponised. Often those holding some of the most destructive weapons don't appear in any images of destruction, because they are creating them. More to the point, 'while some in the video wield hammers, others point cameras, generating new images including the video itself'.

In their acts of destruction, using both hammers and cameras as weapons, ISIS turned the Mosul Museum in Iraq into a new kind of battleground. Beyond these acts of destruction, we are reminded in this book that museums have always been battlegrounds, places where cultures fight over messaging and control. Though there are many who view museums as an unbiased way to learn about the past, museums are far from neutral. They do far more than provide unmediated access to the objects in their collections. Before ISIS and before their attack on the Mosul

Museum, a movement in the museum world was gaining steam: Museums Are Not Neutral. Regardless of what people do who occupy their halls, museums provide a specific framework around the objects they display. Their labels, inherently human in their creation, tell a certain story, one from which bias is impossible to separate.

Contemporary issues of colonialism and repatriation have only served to complicate museum spaces. Tugendhaft writes briefly of attempts by the Iraqi government to reacquire objects from their country's past that are currently housed all over the world in vast colonial institutions like the British Museum and the Louvre. These demands proved futile in a way that Tugendhaft calls 'beside the point'. However, it is worth taking this small anecdote and using it as a way to think more deeply about what it means that Iraqi objects remain outside of Iraq for the most part. While museums are not neutral, they are certainly spaces of control. To, on one hand, have objects in an Iraqi museum destroyed, and on the other hand remain untouched under the influence of American and European museums, introduces an interesting dichotomy. As Tugendhaft points out, to control a museum means to control the representation of a community and how the world perceives it. What many of the world's museums have succeeded in doing is the adoption of the history of Mesopotamia as the foundations of the history of the world. Doing so is the root cause of the worldwide reactions of horror to ISIS's acts of destruction.

Global attention on ISIS's video from within the Mosul Museum was only partially due to the images of destruction. It can be argued that many who reacted with horror did so out of a sense of watching disappear a piece of what has come to be considered cultural heritage of the world. The tendency to identify Mesopotamia as a locus of universal humanity stems from at least the mid-nineteenth century. As the birthplace of so many things that we have come to associate with the civilised world, 'Mesopotamia has come to symbolise what all human beings share'. In today's world of persistent white supremacy, this notion has continued to be problematic. Too often are people willing to adopt the art and writings of ancient Mesopotamia as their own history, while leaving the people of colour responsible for these works and their living ancestors out of the picture.

Though we see a rising wave of white supremacy, it is not by any means a new concept. It was white supremacy in the form of colonialism that drove the first excavations of Assyrian monuments for explorers Émile Botta and Austen Henry Layard. Oft-printed illustrations from their work show these white men standing far above the local workers as they toil in revealing the thousand-pound gypsum monuments. Despite their claims of discovery and the advancement of science, it is images like these that drive home the point that Botta's and Layard's actions were inseparable from nineteenth-century imperial politics. Tugendhaft deftly addresses these issues of colonialism and control, tracing a straight line from initial excavations through to modern museums. In framing these contexts in terms of national prestige, he places ISIS's actions on the same continuum of colonialism, imperialism, and national prestige.

The appropriation of ancient Mesopotamian, specifically Assyrian, imagery has found its way beyond museums and deeper into artistic and political life. For example, many readers will be familiar with the massive winged man that tops Oscar Wilde's tomb in Paris's Père Lachaise cemetery. The sculptor, Jacob Epstein, was inspired by the Assyrian winged bulls, or *lamassu*, that had been recently uncovered at the time of Wilde's death in 1900. Incidentally, many of those dazzling figures can be found in the Louvre, not far from the tomb. As well, the inappropriately named Oriental Institute of the University of Chicago features ancient Assyrian figures as representatives of 'the East' atop the tympanum gracing the building's front door. It is striking to note the presence of these figures alongside the conspicuous absence of any representation of Islam. In the United States and in Europe, the use of these images, while not physically destructive, can be equally damaging in their acceptance of the wonder of the ancient world while maligning the people who occupy the same space today.

Of course, that's not to say that the use of these images in Iraq has been any better or less painful than those already outlined. Like any authoritarian ruler, Saddam Hussein peppered Iraq with images of himself that emphasised both his power and his right to rule via connections to the country's past. Tugendhaft highlights a painted image of Hussein receiving a small palm from an ancient Assyrian man in a way meant to show the transfer of power over thousands of years, culminating with Hussein. The design and deployment of this image was very intentionally filled with references to a glorious ancient past that the current government was very much claiming as its own to justify repressive dictatorial practices. The connections were even present in the language. In Arabic, the word *nachla* means 'palm,' which is the literal object Hussein receives in the image. In Aramaic, one of the languages used in the Assyrian empire, the same word means 'inheritance,' a reference to the power that Hussein is receiving.

Despite the title, this book is not about ISIS, but rather about images. It's about the images we see that deeply affect us, the images we create for a desired effect, and the images we manipulate to serve new means. Using images in these varied and powerful ways is a practice that extends from ancient Assyria, thousands of years ago, through the rediscovery of its ruins, and on to the modern political history of Iraq. Navigating this multitude of ties is certainly a challenge, but one that Tugendhaft handles masterfully in his work. The challenge of *The Idols of ISIS* is to walk away from these stories of image use with a keener eye toward the images that surround us every day.

HISTORICAL MEMORIES

Osama Siddique

Damascus, Baghdad, Basra, Kabul, Herat. That these names mean so little if anything to most contemporary readers is the tragedy. Associated at most with hazy, flickering, granulated images of the latest civil unrest or flashing red lights on modern 3D war maps of the ostensible and perpetual War on Terror. Yet others are either shrouded in the mist of forgetfulness that descended on the post-colonials and took away any clarity of vision about their remote pasts; remain hidden behind an opaqueness inherited from the erstwhile USSR; or are simply less approachable due to various other factors stemming from tyrannies past and present – Lahore, Isfahan, Fes, Samarkand, Bukhara, Cordova, Jerusalem, and many more. Iftikhar Malik's *The Silk Road and Beyond* brings to life and humanises so many of these places that vibrantly exist but are largely invisible to the common gaze.

Divided into three parts, the first is called 'Memoirs' and offers various moving sketches of people and events from the writer's diverse and rich intellectual life – from his sun-drenched village in the picturesque Potohar plateau to his graduate school in cold and snowy Michigan. The final part of the book on the other hand focuses, as the title 'Nestling in the West' indicates, on memorable cultural and intellectual encounters and experiences as a person of, dare I say, Eastern sensibility and Western intellectual rigour. As a matter of fact, this facility of Malik's – painstaking elucidation of complex events and the multiplicity of perspectives on the same, combined with sensitivity and candour while laying bare past and current frameworks for Othering and exploitation of many nations, and particularly the Islamic civilisation – make him an important contemporary scholarly commentator on global history. The middle and longest part of the book is my favourite. It is called 'Traversing the Silk Road' and comprises of twelve chapters on travels in the kind of places that, with some exceptions, are frequently portrayed as obscure and inconsequential nooks of the wider world, if not downright shadowlands, by reductionist segments of the Western media.

Travelling through Bukhara, Samarkand, Tashkent, Jerusalem, Konya, Isfahan, Cordova, Fes and also Pisa and Sicily due to their Islamic connections, Malik skilfully takes on the multiple roles of tourist, historian, commentator and philosopher. These chapters are characterised by detailed but very readable architectural descriptions, cultural insights and succinct capturing of the complex histories of these medieval cities. However, to me what made these accounts additionally meaningful and moving was the deep sense of wistfulness and nostalgia for the past on the part of the author with which they are imbued. On the face of it the journey appears to be an overwhelmingly intellectual one as the author sets out to illuminate the grand history of these metropolises, which lie fairly marginalised in the modern world. Underlining the tremendous past significance of these places he states: 'in Islam's early golden age, cities like Bukhara, Merv, Balkh, Aleppo, Shiraz, Konya, Fes, Cairo, and Baghdad played a vanguard role in spearheading knowledge and arts'. However, it soon transpires that this nostalgia is not purely intellectual; even though the book provides a rich account of the scholars, sages, mystics, scientists, rulers, administrators, artists and writers that populated these lands. This makes the book a valuable resource for anyone wanting to understand and appreciate how these places actually made the so-called dark ages the enlightened ages. What is, therefore, distinctive and somewhat unusual here is the romanticism that permeates the narrative.

Iftikhar H. Malik, *The Silk Road and Beyond: Narratives of a Muslim Historian*, Oxford University Press, Karachi, 2020

Let me elucidate this point. For instance, it is not just the author's commentary on what Bukhara meant for the compilation of Hadith literature and the contribution of Fes to the genesis of degree granting universities, but also his evocative portrayal of their setting, the labyrinthine streets of the old quarters, the vast deserts encircling them, with night caravans progressing from one dimly-lit caravanserai to another in the expired centuries, and the placid yet intellectually abuzz quarters of medieval Muslim teachers, that bring medieval Bukhara and Fes to life and make it such a pleasurable account. While narrating Bukhara's rich intellectual history he of course dwells at length on icons and luminaries like Imam Muhammad Ismail Bukhari, Ibn Sina, Al-Farabi, Al-Biruni, Abu Abdullah Jafar Roudaki, Firdowsi, Al-Khwarizimi, Bahauddin Naqshband, Ulugh Beg and other polymaths and geniuses who either hailed from the city or studied there or spent a formative period in its air that seemed to inspire theological, intellectual and scientific brilliance. However, equally we find history not just being described and analysed but also experienced and felt. Here is an instance of 'feeling' Bukhara rather than merely describing it:

> To me, more than silk and trade, this was the land of Sufis and scholars, long gone to dust but eternalised by their ideas, words, and deeds. So while looking at the houses, madrassas, narrow lanes, austere dwellings made of mud and wooden beams, and the inhabitants, I could not override my sense of history and immersion. I was like the Buddhist monks fresh from Gandhara to reach Sogdiana while the next moment I felt like the Jewish prophets seeking refuge amongst the hospitable people of these tough mountains. And at another level, I also envisioned myself to be a pained soul picking up pieces of my life after one more devastating invasion or an earthquake. Burying the dead and saving my own life while starting all anew was the sum total of my history, as, in my imagination, I would hurry to madrassa to listen to Ibn Sina or relish Firdausi serenading his choicest words to his glorified Persia.

In Fez, the author once more finds himself transported by the medieval feel of the place and urges the readers to join him in his imaginative journey:

> Fez or Fes, the Fesians prefer the latter, is certainly an overwhelming place where, in its old Medina, time seems to have stopped a long time ago, and where modernity sheepishly stands aloof as a curious observer and not like a hegemon. Except for electricity and mobile phones, it does not seem to have made any difference to this great medieval city. Like its other compatriots in Marrakesh, Rabat, Sale, and Meknes, Fes is a rare place on earth where one is pliantly transferred back into the Medieval Ages. At night, it is even more mysterious, majestic, and observant as if both time and history had come to an absolute stop. If one ignores the street bulbs, a few zealous shopkeepers, or

> some happily lost tourists with a sweaty pink glow, Fez is still catholically pre-modern and must stay so.

At the same time, the book is of salience not just for its engagement with the more known historical figures but even more so for the lesser familiar figures it brings to attention. Such as the dynamic sisters from Fes, that remains one of the oldest, biggest and best-preserved medieval cities in the world. Here he introduces us to the famous mosque and madrassa of Karaouine and to these sisters:

> In Karaouine, Ibn Rushd, Maimonides, and Ibn Khaldun taught at the world's oldest degree awarding university as it had been housed in one of the biggest mosques in the Muslim world, watched over by two minarets that were replicated in Marrakesh, Rabat and Seville. The mosque and the madrassa were established by Fatima al-Fihiri in 859 CE, who herself was a refugee from Kairouan in present day Tunisia. Her sister, Mariam founded a mosque across the river Jawhar for displaced Andalusian Muslims, and in between these two historic institutions stands the Sidi Ahmed al-Tijani Madrassa founded for African Muslims.

Fatima al-Fihri and Mariam al-Fihri – what absolutely remarkable persons they must have been. Visionary, pioneering and enterprising by the standards of any age, but especially so, so far back in the distant ninth century, and doubly so given the constraints and challenges posed by their gender that continue to acutely inhibit many women even a millennia later. Founders of mosques and madrassas and perhaps so much more that lay the foundation of a glorious intellectual tradition, centuries before the emergence of such continuing centres of learning in the West. Yet they remain names obscure to most, and especially to the latest representatives and inheritors of their civilisation. By placing and highlighting them in the very heart of the intellectual and cultural ferment of which they were a part, Malik coaxes us to shed our ignorance and prejudices and to recognise and celebrate such glorious aspects of the past free from the debilitating myopia of the present.

Malik has a bold craving to excavate the signs of, and rediscover, a span of time during the medieval era which is regarded by many as a Golden Period of Islam. When, as he says,

> sacred and secular existed in comparative harmony anchoring what Professor Mohammed Arkoun (1928-2010) calls Global Humanism. Their political, intellectual, scientific, and cultural accomplishments ensured a greater sense of self-confidence and tolerance towards non-Muslims. The contemporary world of Islam had a sense of belonging to a dynamic global civilisation despite its varying metropolitan centres such as the Abbasids in Baghdad, the Fatimids in North Africa and Sicily, the Arab-Berber-Spanish Caliphate in Spain, Ismailis in Khorasan and north-western India, and the Seljuks in Asia Minor. Here the imperial pursuits converged with faith even if they might embody factionalism, yet entrepreneurship, literary, and artistic achievements, and openness towards the world at large underwrote their collective ethos.

It ought to be acknowledged, however, that Malik's preoccupation is not exclusively with the past. He is also someone who fully appreciates the contemporary and relishes and appreciates whatever of value it has to offer. His account is full of his enthusiastic and often joyful engagement with the cities he visits and their populace. Yet he also lifts the curtains and provides us vivid and impactful glimpses of what these grand cities would have looked and felt like in years gone by, the glory and the travails that they encountered, their interconnectedness through commercial and intellectual routes, and their tremendous contributions to human civilisation. Through his sensitive and careful portrayal of the thought and knowledge production in these medieval powerhouses, he endeavors to lay bare and fling aside dehumanised and distorted representations of their past and present. Thereby he reweaves significant linkages with the past that are not just essential for an informed, enriched and much more-self-assured modern Islamic identity but also a tolerant and global universal identity. A tolerant and global universal identity that avoids misleading and destructive demarcations, divides and clashes envisioned by the champions of 'Clash of Civilisation'; that embraces all that is of value, regardless of where it stems from, in order to enrich and contribute to a collective human civilisational project.

The Silk Road and Beyond is a delightful and informative read for anyone interested in this fascinating region as well as seeking a crisp analytical summation of their history over the middle ages. At the same time, it is a contemporary travelogue that captures the sights and sounds of these colourful and majestic cities and demystifies Western popular misconceptions. In addition to being an eminent historian with a vast array of interests, Malik has particular interest in art and architecture and thus there is much here that would interest art and architecture enthusiasts. With passion and obvious pride Malik excavates and brings to attention the cosmopolitanism, plurality, tolerance and love of knowledge that thrived and continues to thrive in the many cultures that collectively form the Muslim civilisation. There is no timidity and sense of apology here as the fetishes of past exoticisation and even demonisation of these cultures is taken head on and contested for their disingenuity. Considered and nuanced in what he chooses to describe, discuss and analyse, Malik offers a compelling blend of history, travel and memoire.

ET CETERA

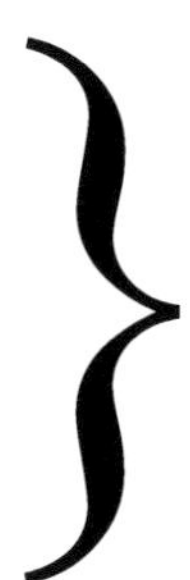

LAST WORD

ON COGNITIVE IMMUNITY

Ebrahim Moosa

Humans and microbes are interdependent. Humans are often the hosts, but so too are animals, plants and nature generally. In the main, these relationships are beneficial and harmless. Our dependence on microbes is critical to our own survival such as the bacteria in our gut.

But some microbes are viruses. These microbes require hosts – humans, animals and plants – in order to unleash their damaging, and, sometimes lethal power. It is the supreme parasite with a difference: it carries information in its core make-up in the form of DNA and RNA and then gains intelligibility in the host. And then like every intruder it creates havoc in the body. Machines can also be affected by cyber viruses. Their subversive information codes can jam up entire networks and impact the lives of millions. Cyber viruses can even penetrate lethal nuclear reactors and could accidentally set off nuclear accidents or precipitate cyber as well as other forms of warfare.

Once a virus' genetic composition unravels into the body or the cyber virus hacks the network, then things literally go haywire. Like hay held together by clumsy wire, hence the term 'haywire', the body or the machine gets tied down, becomes dysfunctional for a duration until a repair can be made. Most times this invasion passes through the body or is reversed. But some viruses, like the Covid-19 virus, come armed with a spike and tentacles which debilitate the body's cells and disables it from performing its proper function, often with fatal consequences. But thanks to our advancement in biology and epidemiology we have a fairly good picture of pathogens and have found vaccines to immunise ourselves against such invaders. Yet, our latest encounter with viruses at pandemic levels allows us to ponder and reflect on several points.

We have come a long way since a time when we did not have the foggiest idea of what it specifically was about putrid conditions and squalor that impacted human health. The Black Death in the mid 1300s took millions of lives. Improved epidemiology, sanitation and monoclonal antibodies that mimic the body's capacity to fight off harmful viruses are major pharmacological interventions along the way.

Prior to our detailed knowledge of pathogens, early societies had to monitor the symptoms produced in the body and fight off the unknown agents and their symptoms. Hellenic medicine and its followers among Jewish, Christian and Muslim physicians over time grasped the causes of illness. At a very early stage in this account of our knowledge of pathogens and disease, physicians relied on cosmological auguries to determine health and illness. Earthly conditions were mapped to movements and alignments in the heavens and our relationships to the locations of planets and stars. Astrology played a critical role in informing medical theory. One such author was Kūshyār Ibn Labbān (971–1029), a Persian mathematician and astronomer. In an introduction to astrology Ibn Labbān identifies diseases in relation to the motions of the moon. Human bodies were associated with certain astral types and times. Medicines and remedies found sympathies and antipathies with certain body types. Outbreaks of diseases and illnesses and the recovery from disease could also be predicted from astral times.

But there were also physicians like the famous Ibn Sīnā (980–1037) who explored material causes for disease. Epidemics were associated with widescale fevers among population groups. Interestingly, Ibn Sīnā in his famous book *The Canon in Medicine* writes about fevers stemming from contagion and infectious diseases. When describing epidemics, he speaks mostly about the role of weather conditions and patterns like winds and environmental conditions that facilitate contagion. Contagion, he explained, stemmed from the contamination of the water supply, but primarily the contamination of the air followed by its effects on the body. Today most of us understand this phenomenon as the viral load in a given space, thanks to our most recent experience with the Covid-19 virus and the global pandemic in its wake in 2020 and our awareness that viruses largely spread through aerosol particles.

So, even in the annals of Muslim history there were different approaches to disease and different diagnoses of their causes. While these different approaches to medicine in the past might appear irreconcilable, we possess insufficient social history of those periods to reach any categorical conclusions. Yet one wishes if only a modicum of such historical literacy survived in communities around the world so that we could avoid falling foul of conspiracy theories and in the process abandon structured judgment to further epidemiological and medical remedies.

One lesson this pandemic taught is the need for humans to combat comorbidities and to optimise one's bodily immunity. If unfulfilled, then an unhealthy body will allow for all kinds of chronic diseases to set in and then our bodies will become magnets for parasitical invaders.

In times of crisis too all kinds of half-baked and grandiose ideas float around on social media posturing as knowledge and then these ideas literally 'go viral', a term used in marketing and by advertisers. Instead of manufacturers and producers investing time and money to market their products, the end-users and customers do the marketing. Products become so alluring that customers believe other people should also have them, ranging from social media apps to electronic gadgets to fashion. If this is the rationale for enticing the public to alluring goods and foods such as named coffee brands to jeans and clothing lines, then the same kind of logic would also apply to things that people find repulsive such as the use of animal furs, anti-animal-abuse campaigns and the targeted boycott of goods and services. Living in the viral lane of life fosters push-button decision-making that seeks instant gratification without sufficient reflection and contemplation associated with both. As much as social media can be helpful in the circulation of ideas and mobilising people, it also has a downside.

One downside of the social media generation and living in the viral lane is that it impacts cognitive immunity. Impaired cognitive immunity can result in harmful social outcomes. Marina Gorbis and Nick Monaco argue that healthy cognitive immunity is a pre-requisite for democracy. Often advocates or critics living in the viral lane do not spend sufficient time to see the merit in an idea or a product they disapprove of nor can they see the demerits in things they approve. Living on social media and in the viral lane, can result in viral overload and cognitive poverty. As

Gorbis writes: 'to upgrade our cognitive immune system we need to recognise the complex system of technologies, institutional arrangements, beliefs, individual predispositions, and many other factors that shape social cognition and activate multiple levers. We call these levers "immunity activators"'.

In a span of less than a year cognitive vulnerability spiked during the pandemic. Not truth, but rather thinking became the pandemic's first casualty. How many WhatsApp messages did you not receive in 2020 about the diabolical people behind the Covid-19 virus. Everyone from China to the billionaire Bill Gates were culpable for the pandemic. And those opposed to vaccines, the antivaxxers, have spun endless fabrications about the effect of the anti-Covid-19 vaccines on the human body.

In an environment where we are habituated to memes and virally-traded products, especially in the realms of news and information, it is precisely where cognitive immunity is at its lowest and most vulnerable. Rational argument can hardly make a breakthrough since people are hooked onto beliefs. Note the reluctance, nay refusal, of millions around the world to follow public health protocols during the pandemic that could have saved thousands of human lives. US President Donald Trump mastered the art of viral marketing of his own brand of politics, namely lies, deceit and bluster. But he managed to convince tens of millions from among the 70 million people who voted for him in the 2020 presidential elections. Many believe that the voting process was rigged without a shred of compelling evidence. By falsifying the truth about the US elections, Trump and the politicians who supported him, fomented an insurrection resulting in a violent mob storming the US Capitol on 6 January 2021.

Thinking, reason and logic have become orphaned despite enhanced literacy around the world. A more thorough diagnosis as to why irrationality increases with a growth in literacy is needed. Moderns prize the fact that science drives a large part of our civilisation. Everything from transportation, communications and all industries from agriculture, medicine, education, entertainment to protecting the environment now come under some authority of science and technology. We built a global civilisation in all these domains, wrote American astrophysicist and popular science writer, Carl Sagan and we 'profoundly depend on science and technology'. But he also sounded a warning that we fully experienced in

2020 with the large-scale disregard for science around the world. 'We have also arranged things', said Sagan, 'so that almost no one understands science and technology'. 'This is a prescription for disaster', he added. 'We might get away with it for a while, but sooner or later this combustible mixture of ignorance and power is going to blow up in our faces,' Sagan warned in 1996. Nearly a quarter century later we experienced what he predicted almost to the letter.

During the Covid-19 pandemic, the level of disregard for scientific insight was astounding. Large numbers of ordinary people from different political and religious persuasions, heads of government, professionals of all stripes ignored science with fatal consequences. At the time of writing nearly 1.5 million people died globally as a direct result of the pandemic. So one take home is that the virus does not only strike those with underlying conditions but also impacts those who lack cognitive immunity. Many people who disregard public health warnings get infected and transmit it to others. With the large-scale environmental crisis already inescapable, Sagan might yet be right: things are already blowing up in our faces but we are unable to sufficiently recognise it.

Another way of describing impaired cognitive immunity is to consider people's inability to be viewed as figurative mental viruses. Entire communities find their cognitive immunity being hijacked by internet trolls to the point that folks are unable to distinguish fact from fiction. One result is that increasingly people around the world demonstrate the lack of a shared understanding of facts and realities. These are beyond cultural differences. Vaccines are deemed a hoax and a desperate effort by pharmaceutical companies to fleece humanity. Drug companies are viewed as the shock troops of capitalism to hook us into drug and medicine dependency. Pharmaceutical companies have a lot to answer for, but are life-saving vaccines one of them?

A large number of people around the world believe that the deaths and destruction caused in New York and Washington on 11 September 2001 by terrorists were events that never truly happened as we saw it. The World Trade Center buildings were not destroyed by jetliners but rather the US government caused a controlled demolition of the structure in order to justify their pre-planned invasion of Afghanistan and Iraq in a bid to destroy the emerging possibilities of Muslim ways of life and caliphal governance reaching fruition. Few people know that the slick documentaries supporting the 9/11 conspiracy were made by professional conspiracy theorists and right-wing groups, among them Alex Jones. Denialists of all kinds will have ready-made answers and superficially rationally-sounding counter rhetoric. It ceases to be a rational conversation because there is no shared understanding of the facts under consideration, nor do people agree on the facts. Impaired cognitive immunity has metastasised on a global scale and engulfed rich and poor nations alike. One is reminded of a popular rhyming Arabic proverb: madness comes in multiple art forms (*li ʾl-junūn funūn*).

Perversion of the truth is not a new phenomenon but perhaps we might be noticing it more frequently given the extraordinary effective forms of monitoring and global media as well as social media traffic at our disposal. Already in the nineteenth century, the novelist Fyodor Dostoevsky grasped this penchant to distort reality. 'Man has such a predilection for systems and abstract deductions that he is ready to distort the truth intentionally he is ready to deny the evidence of his senses only to justify his logic'.

In her aptly titled book for our times *Contagious*, Priscilla Wald discusses social contagion, a term derived from sociological, bacteriological, and epidemiological research as an emerging conception of community formation. The French man of letters Gustave Le Bon, she tells us, deployed the concept of contagion in his popular study, *The Crowd: A Study of the Popular Mind*, when it was published in 1885. It commonly describes how an individual gets 'caught up in the spirit and actions of a group, surrendering personal agency and even rational thought to the collective will'. Contagion aptly describes populism gone berserk in the USA under the banner of Trumpism, as well as in Brazil, Hungary and in India, to mention a few places. Le Bon anatomised crowds, which he likened to 'those microbes which hasten the dissolution of enfeebled or dead bodies'. Contagion is the effect of suggestibility and enables crowds to emerge irrationally and without forethought, writes Wald. She documents how the outbreak narratives invoke the language of warfare. For a few days, Donald Trump, momentarily cast himself as a war president in battle against the Covid-19 virus but then quietly dropped the appellation once he failed at finding a strategy to combat and stem the epidemiological crisis.

Wald's insights, and our recent experience with Covid-19-related deaths, all confirm her conclusions that the exclusive focus on biomedical treatment, in fact, masks the important role socioeconomic factors play in health outcomes. In the US, at least, the economically poor and racially marginalised were disproportionately affected in both Covid-19-related deaths and illnesses, although the affluent sectors too were affected. Around the world the most vulnerable are exposed to the virus but we still do not have reliable statistics regarding mortality rates in proportion to economic status.

If we have learned anything from the Covid-19 pandemic then it has taught us that our vulnerability to viruses might radically increase in the future, especially pathogens transmitted from animals to humans due to environmental stress and other pressures. Varieties of viruses are going to be our long-term companions. We might get better at finding solutions to such pestilential invaders over shorter durations given advances in microbiology and gene-based therapies. If we wish to keep the mortality rates down during such future afflictions then bodily as well as cognitive immunity are prerequisites.

TEN LESSONS FROM THE PANDEMIC

A wonderful video went viral on social media a couple months into the global lockdown. Fantastical music plays as a father reads one last story to his son before he drifts off into a slumber of peaceful dreams. The tale tells of a far off and hypothetical land that was ravaged by climate devastation, by poverty and excess, with limitless growth, wants, and instant gratification. Where talking continued but meaning and social bonds were lost. A world where minor imperfections were filtered out with their technology and everyone become complacent in their unerring loneliness. In their search for wonder, the planet was destroyed. But then a virus came along, an invisible enemy, that forced all the people to hide. When they hid, the people learned to appreciate the small things, appreciate the planet, find their meaning, and learn to love each other again. As the father concluded the story, the son perked up to say, 'but why did it take a virus to bring the people back together?' The father replies with a smile: 'sometimes you've got to get sick my boy, before you start feeling better.'

Now, after experiencing the impact of the pandemic, we can reflect and critique a year with the virus. The Covid-19 pandemic has changed things (whether or not it will 'change everything' remains to be seen). But we still have three options before us. Change for the better, change for the worst, and, perhaps worst of all, change nothing. While 'post-' has become a clichéd prefix of late, what words it will precede remains to be seen and will depend on the actions taken at the present. Perhaps, we will hear less of postmodernism, postcolonialism, and even move beyond the post-9/11 world. But will the post-Covid world be any better?

Hopefully, one day we can look back on this all in the past tense. Meanwhile, here are a few lessons from the year the Earth stood still. Perhaps hindsight will indeed prove to be 20/20. Take heed so that history need not repeat itself for those who were not listening!

1. Which jobs are indeed essential to society (thank you, grocery delivery folks!)

When governments around the globe first started to enact movement restrictions, it appeared for a moment that the end-of-the-world nuts may have had it right. But thankfully we didn't all need to stock pile munitions or learn to grow or hunt for our own food. We owe an innumerable debt to the front liners, the real heroes who taught us what are indeed the essential services needed. Interestingly enough, these were not heads of state, CEOs, executives, or the financial gurus who hold the majority of the planet's wealth. It is instead those we pay, and otherwise often treat, the worst in our societies. Perhaps we all will now go forward with a greater appreciation for those who keep our groceries stocked, our parcels moving from one point to the next, the bank tellers, the tradesmen who keep the electricity and WIFI coming in and the rubbish and loo evacuations going out, the healthcare workers who have quite literally risked life and limb over the past year, and everyone else we would not bat an eye over until they are truly gone and suddenly we are forced back to the dark ages. As we cheer for them today, let us not forget to carry forward that appreciation into tomorrow. We need to take note of the fact that society is a collective and that it takes all of us doing our part to keeping its functioning and moving. We thank those who have risked it all to keep it all spinning, and those who could, for staying in and practicing good healthcare policy. When we can say that it is all over, let us not forget those who keep the great machine churning.

2. And that effective governance is not as essential as we had hoped...

Few governments around the globe will go without poor marks on their Covid response report cards, but some of the worst offenders are the supposed mega-democracies which hail themselves to be the bastions of virtue! The US, the UK, India, and Brazil have topped the Covid case and death ratings month after month. But perhaps the veneer of democracy is giving way to older and more dangerous social factors. The divisions that exist all around the world in numerous societies have been commonly trending towards a breaking point and while this can reflect in the poor track records of some of the largest countries in the world, one of the greatest revelations in recent times is the compounding of contradictions and problems with what was normal before the virus. While movement restriction did, for a moment, quell the civil unrest from East to West, it was not long before political unrest re-emerged, even if, in some cases, it had to move to the digital sphere. Prior to and continuing strong throughout lockdowns, political crises remain and are near boiling point in Hong Kong, Thailand, the US, Belarus, Malaysia, India, France, Poland, Nigeria and many other places. But there is one more lesson to be learned for future governance. Is it surprising that some of the best Covid responses come from countries led by women? From Jacinda Ardern in New Zealand to Tsai Ing-wen in Taiwan to the numerous female leaders in Europe, women have been getting the job done and keeping the ship afloat! Female leadership is also driving grass-roots and resistance movements from the US to Ecuador, Poland, Nigeria, and throughout Asia. If things are going to change, it is good to see some of the young changers becoming political.

3. That everyone is self-centred, yet each paragons of our own independent virtue!

But inspiring the masses can be difficult and we can't all be Damilola Odufuwa and Odunayo Eweniyi of Nigeria or Poland's Klementyna Suchanow. So why not take a quick selfie, jump on social media and form a cult of yourself. And after all, who knows better than me? And look how bad everyone else is, and who knows best which movements to get behind or which tragedies to sympathise with? And when has my Facebook feed ever steered me wrong? Since World War II, individualism has been on a rapid rise, particularly in the West but thanks to globalised popular culture it can be for everyone! And while Margaret Thatcher would be spinning in her grave over the amount of Covid relief being handed out by governments around the world, the showrunners of Netflix's *The Crown* would hope the audience should be cringing as Gillian Anderson, portraying the Iron Lady, recited the infamous 'there is no society, there are only individuals'. But do our actions agree more than we would like with such sentiments. In our isolation, a certain narcissism seems to take control when escapism is no longer possible and we take stock of our present condition. Social media has quickly continued its tendency to be a place to 'look at me' as oppose to maintain social communication. Those crying for rights, care less about the common welfare than their own comfort from demanding free speech to resisting the tyranny of facemasks. *Vive la liberté*! We shall see what good that does if there are none of us around to enjoy it.

4. That we really have no idea how far 6 feet (or 2 metres) is

For a vast majority of us it is difficult to judge measurement (depth perception notwithstanding). That's why we have measuring tape, but to keep you from having to add another survival item to lug around during out-of-home excursions, many governments and organisations have taken advantage of our ability to use measurement by analogy. So, the recommended social distance is an average person's arm span, five escalators steps, a twin size bed mattress, or half of one Volkswagen Beetle. How has your public performance measured? Adapting to these new procedures is difficult, but it is a willingness to socially distance, properly wash up, and don the facemask that demonstrates that we have learned the lesson about selfishness. After all, these regulations actually do the very minimum to protect you directly, as by going outside you are engaging with the world and left with a Schrödinger's Cat question about what is and is not infected. But by wearing a mask and social distancing, more importantly you are significantly decreasing your ability to pass on anything you have picked up out there in the world. Indeed, a mask does not have to be political statement, but it can be a symbol of humanism and love for one's neighbour. And for those of you whom a digital hug just does not seem to have the same effect, here is a literary hug. I am not sure if that helped, but at least we are amply socially distanced.

5. Working at home in pyjamas can be highly productive and comfortable!

During the pandemic traditional notions of human productivity, its ups and downs, have been redefined. It is amazing what people can accomplish when they can be comfortable. And to think, all the time saved, having to get up and prim and prime one's self for the day ahead. Why even get out of your pyjamas? When you're working from home, there is no need to craft one's hair or put on any make-up. Keep it cosy and let the mind open up to new and smart ways to get the day's workload accomplished. Who needs the day-to-day pressure of having to care what other's think of your appearance? Break whenever you want, grab a snack, a tea, or a coffee, use the toilet without having to let anyone know or have anyone cover for you. Calls and emails ought to be kept up on, but it's pandemic days and no one really needs anything *immediately*. So, if a lunchbreak turns into a full Netflix series binge session, *hakuna matata*, you can make sure to put in the extra effort tomorrow. And why not change things up? You can work from a different part of the house each day, or even try opening a window and getting fresh air, or working in the garden. And if you need to catch a quick Zoom meeting, then throw on a nice shirt and whip your hair back and forth and trouser liberation enthusiasts the world over rejoice! Just make sure to turn off your camera if you need to get up for a drink refill. But what's that, the kids need to be entertained? That construction next door feels like they are in my living room with me! Dinner needs to be made? Your partner is typing or thinking too loudly. Whose been slacking on the chores? When was the last time we took out the rubbish? When was the last time you showered? This one goes out to the pandemic parents who have to both keep their kids and selves on track and to you who finally read that book (or even written that book) that you'd been promising you'd read (or write) if you just had a little more time. Our condolences to those who's workloads blew up this year.

6. But motivation is not guaranteed by Amazon Prime

While the pandemic and lockdown have left many of us with a considerable surplus of time this year, the same cannot always be said for motivation. When one is not physically required to 'get out of bed' how can the same be expected mentally. Being required to stay in is taxing and numerous studies have shown that solitary confinement is unnatural to human beings, nigh inhumane, in line with torture. To cope, many of us treat these days as if nothing had changed, maintain the routine and even dress as if going to work, to then sit at one corner of the home and get cracking. Others have taken on various wellness techniques from frequent breaking to taking on meditation or yoga. In our taking on the reality of the world in confinement we have leaned heavily on personal treats and the safe convenience that technology offers. Since we cannot go out, then we order and let us be thankful for the gig economy army that allows us to move items to and fro and even ourselves if needed with minimal risk and maximum convenience. With those who lost their jobs during the pandemic, the gig economy has been a wonderful way for people to secure their incomes and keep themselves and their families afloat during this trying time. But with that, we must ask, what is the other side of the coin? Amazon and other online retailers are making record profits, but it is well known that this new wealth does not in fact trickle down to those out there 'in it'. And since the gig economy offers little in the way of protections, security, and pension as the traditional workforce, who is looking out for them? Yet, with more time, the true innovative and entrepreneurial spirits of others have been allowed to blossom, whether that is starting a career as a YouTube celebrity or finding a way to use technology to your advantage when human-to-human contact is to be avoided. The pros and cons pile up and yet the lessons to be learned may not be visible until well after the pandemic.

7. *Proper use of your mute button and digital backgrounds have become survival skills*

Zoom was one of over a dozen other major group chat applications that came into their own. Through a magic not unknown to the Silicon Valley world, Zoom rose to the top through network popularity while pouring its resources into servers so that it has plenty of space for high volumes of users. Zooming became a word in 2020 and is almost as big as Googling. Thanks to having a free option and an easy-to-use interface, Zoom is the digital space of choice, but with any new technological step, comes a bit of a learning curve. Where the chimes of a mobile used to be the most disruptive potential during a class or meeting (and honestly this has somewhat numbed in our 24/7, interconnected world) hell hath no fury like the death scares and annoyance over a random noise from an unmuted attendee interrupting a speaker. Likewise, an unspoken competition has arisen concerning backgrounds. You will be judged by the books on the shelf behind you, so chose wisely. On the news, one must assert their political allegiance with the cannons of liberal or conservative literature or nationalism through flags and hanging merits. If you cannot compete, then chose from the default digital backgrounds, or be so bold as to download your own. Who says dazzling green screen technological feats are only for *Star Wars* films? Just remember to check your speaker and camera settings, lest you let an inappropriate viewing or noise be broadcast to your digital friends!

8. A pandemic is a nice, new, excuse for not being able to get down to the gym

New Year's resolutions from 2020 may have been given a pass in light of Covid-19, but will we all be so lucky in 2021? We were amazed how many people ran to the beaches during the momentary breaks in lockdown that 2020 saw, after all, we all know lockdown does not bode well for the ideal beach bod. After the first month of lockdown, it became apparent to many that this was going to be one for the long haul and if we did not get creative about our activity, a whole host of other issues lie in waiting, not to mention how tragic it would be for the world not to see your most recent post-workout selfie! A flurry of videos and at-home workout plans rose in popularity as many struggle to maintain their form. Even some who had not been regular exercisers found a needed escape in being able to get active, be that purchasing a treadmill or other exercise equipment, or even going for a walk or bicycle ride when allowed. Zoom made for another way for trainers to keep at work and host classes and sessions to vast numbers of people all over the world. While gymnasiums were hit hard by lockdowns, after deep cleaning and ensuring a safe standard operating procedure, they quickly filled up to the half capacities they were allowed. Facemask designers were faced with the unenviable task of creating a protective, yet comfortable facemask that allowed people to push themselves physically without having to suffer from the limitations put upon by masking up. With a mix of proper social distancing and, dare we say, rather fashionable facemasks, the new normal leaves us with no excuse for not getting that daily exercise.

9. Clean air is possible, and quite refreshing too!

As lockdowns killed airline and automotive travel, a noticeable cut back in pollution clouds prompted the trending of #EarthIsHealing. Distant sights once hidden by pollution haze were again becoming visible, water was returning to a recognisable blue hue, and even certain animals began taking back the habitat that human growth had impeded upon. Not to mention the noise pollution cutbacks too! Species on the verge, even a few thought long gone, were spotted again in places that living memory could hardly recall. For a moment we were cut off and nature was allowed to do what it does best, uninhibited. And it was nice to breath clean air and not be choked by industrial smells. Maybe we have been given a wakeup call on climate change, maybe we can change and perhaps there is even still time for us to change. But we need to think long and hard about how we come back from the pandemic. Let us hope a new age of ecological consciousness, or at least a greater appreciation for living with the natural world, has been awoken in our isolation.

10.We really need to be talking about mental health issues and other crises

Millions of people all around the world have lost their jobs (which to many were also their livelihood) due to Covid-19.This statistic doesn't begin to encompass the true scale of impact that the pandemic has had on our lives. Work reduction, delays of payment, interruption of supply chains and communication. Humans are also social creatures. Not being able to see our friends, family, and even the random people we bump into as we go about our everyday trajectories. The global halt, the new normal. All of this adaptation, change, and disruption. We all deal with it in different ways and more than we care to admit have reached various breaking points. The trend of deteriorating mental health has been on the steady increase long before Covid-19. Modernity, capitalism, politics, society have all contributed their fair share to this growing crisis. Our brains are only able to deal with so much at once. And the normal ways we used to deal with the world have been drastically limited lately. We need to be talking about mental health and tearing down taboos that keep others from seeking help when it is truly needed. While it is difficult to pin down, due both to reporting and recognition problems, most authorities agree suicide rates have drastically increased during the Covid-19 pandemic. But the need for creative and innovative reform of mental health thinking is a long time coming. Now that the pandemic helps us focus in on this crisis, we can also see the simultaneous compounding of other crises from economic, to political, refugees, climate, epistemological, personal, identity, and so many more all weighing down on us. And if mental health is out, then that's the endgame that is truly sobering.

While we need to keep laughing, so that we are not crying, it is essential we take these lessons to heart. Let's not do this again anytime soon.

CITATIONS

Introduction: Virus Chronicles by Ehsan Masood

Michael Rosen told *The Guardian* how his brush with covid felt like "pre-death": https://www.theguardian.com/books/2020/sep/30/michael-rosen-on-his-covid-19-coma-it-felt-like-a-pre-death-a-nothingness. Nature's news teams began tracking the virus from the start of January. The first three months of coverage is here: https://www.nature.com/articles/d41586-020-00154-w. Why bats harbour so many viruses: https://www.nytimes.com/2020/01/28/science/bats-coronavirus-Wuhan.html. The first of many reports from Imperial College London's Covid-19 monitoring team warned the world in mid-January 2020 that the virus was much more virulent than first thought: https://www.imperial.ac.uk/mrc-global-infectious-disease-analysis/covid-19/report-1-case-estimates-of-covid-19/. The World Health Organization's timeline of events and the agency's responses to events: https://www.who.int/emergencies/diseases/novel-coronavirus-2019/interactive-timeline. The WHO in 2015 issued guidance on the naming of new infectious diseases: https://www.who.int/news/item/08-05-2015-who-issues-best-practices-for-naming-new-human-infectious-diseases. 'The Biomedical Bubble' from science policy researchers James Wilsdon and Richard Jones shows how a developed country such as the UK can spend very large amounts of money on biomedical science, without prioritizing its public health: https://www.nesta.org.uk/report/biomedical-bubble/. An update (as of the end of November 2020) on which countries have secured coronavirus vaccines: https://www.nature.com/articles/d41586-020-03370-6. The Wellcome Trust, one of the world's largest biomedical funding agencies, has been monitoring the state of vaccine hesitancy around the world: https://wellcome.org/reports/wellcome-global-monitor/2018/chapter-5-attitudes-vaccines. Michael Rosen's poem; J'accuse, can be read here: http://michaelrosenblog.blogspot.com/2020/12/jaccusea-government-of-not-protecting-us.html

Justice for a Praying Person by Anwar Ibrahim

Al-Fatani's Munyatul Musalli is available in original Malay and various translations, and extracts from the book, as well discussion on its contents, can be heard on YouTube. For a more elaborated discussion, see Wan Mohd Shaghir Abdullah, *Mun-Yatul Mushalli*

Syeikh Daud Abdullah al-Fathani: Pengetahuan Sembahyang Masyhur (Khazanah Fathaniah, Kuala Lumpur, 1991).

The western works referred to in this essay include: Dante Alighieri *The Divine Comedy* (Everyman's Library, London, 1995), John Donne, *The Complete English Poems* (Penguin, London, 1977), Ernest Hemingway, *For Whom the Bell Tolls* (Scribner, New York, 1995), John Steinbeck's *East of Eden* (Viking, New York, 2003), Plato, *Republic* (Cambridge University Press, Cambridge, 2012), John Locke, *Second Treatise on Government* (Hackett, Indianapolis, 1980), Thomas Hobbes, *Leviathan* (Penguin Classics, London, 1982), Jean Jacques Rousseau, *The Social Contract* (Penguin Classics, London, 1968), John Stewart Mill, *Utilitarianism* (Hackett, Indianapolis, 2002), John Rawls, *The Theory of Justice* (Belknap, Cambridge, 2005), Robert Nozick, *Anarchy, State, and Utopia* (Basic Books, New York, 2013), and Amartya Sen, *The Idea of Justice* (Belknap, Cambridge, 2009).

The following works of Islamic philosophy are mentioned: Abu Nasr Al-Farabi, *On the Perfect Sate*, translated by Richard Walzer (Kazi, Chicago, 1998), Ibn Rushd, Tahafut Al-Tahafut, translated by Simon Van Den Bergh (EJW Gibb Memorial Trust, London, 1978, two volumes), Khaled Abou El Fadl, *Reasoning with God: Reclaiming Shari'ah in the Modern Age* (Rowman & Littlefield, Lanham, 2014), Mohammad Hashim Kamali, *Freedom, Equality and Justice in Islam* (Islamic Text Society, Kuala Lumpur, 2002), and Syed Muhammad Naquib Al-Attas, *On Justice and The Nature of Man* (IBFIM, Kuala Lumpur, 2015).

Also mentioned: Marshall G Hodgson, *The Venture of Islam* (University of Chicago Press, 1974, four volumes); Ziauddin Sardar and Jeremy Henzell-Thomas's *Rethinking Reform in Higher Education: From Islamization to Integration of Knowledge* (IIIT, Herndon, 2017); and Ziauddin Sardar, 'The Erasure of Islam', *The Philosopher's Magazine* 42 (3) 77-79 2008, his quote on the Enlightenment is taken from this article.

For more on Chinese Philosophy and East-West comparative philosophy see: Roger T. Ames, *The Analects of Confucius: A Philosophical Translation* (Ballantine Books, New York, 1999), *Sun Tzu: The Art of War* (Ballantine Books, New York, 1993), David A. Hall and Roger T. Ames, *Anticipating China: Thinking Through the Narratives of Chinese and Western Culture* (SUNY, New York, 1995), and Osman Bakar and Cheng Gek Nai, *Islam and Confucianism: A Civilizational Dialogue* (University of Malaya Press, Kuala Lumpur, 1997).

On John Rawl's comeback, see Julian Coman, 'Can liberalism's great philosopher ride to the west's recue again?' *The Observer* 20 December 2020, pp52-53, which can be read at the Guardian UK website. For more on Postnormal Times, see: *The Postnormal Times Reader* edited by Ziauddin Sardar (IIIT, London, 2019) and www.postnormaltim.es

The Metaphysics of Viruses by Colin Tudge

Rachel Nuwer' blog, 'Why the world needs viruses to function' is on BBVC Future (18 June 2020): https://www.bbc.com/future/article/20200617-what-if-all-viruses-disappeared

Colin Tudge's book *Why Genes are Not Selfish and People are Nice* is published by Floris Books, Edinburgh, 2013. See also: Karl Popper, *Unended Quest*, Routledge Classics, London, 2002.

From God to God by Syed Nomanul Haq

I must acknowledge my debt to Michael Dols. I have drawn rather heavily upon his many seminal studies of the history of plague in Muslim societies. In particular, I have been guided by his "Plague in Early Islamic History" (*Journal of the American Oriental Society*, Vol. 94, No. 3, 1974); "The Comparative Communal Responses to the Black Death in Muslim and Christian Societies" (*Viator*. Vol. 5, 1974. I have followed the pagination of the Stanford version of this essay); and *The Black Death in the Middle East* (Princeton NJ: Princeton University Press, 1977). The verses quoted as the proem of this article is from Ibn 'Asākir's Ta'rīkh Dimashq (Damascus, AH 1332, Vol. 1) quoted in Dols, "Plague in Early Islamic History," pp. 377-78). The 'Amwās story of Abū 'Ubayda appears in the *Badhl* of Ibn Ḥajar al-'Asqalanī quoted in Dols, "Plague in Early Islamic History," p. 377.

The three Hadith reports are from the *Book of Medicine* of the canonical Bukhari. The reports have standardized numbering, even though there are many standardizations. I have used the website <https://sunnah.com/bukhari/76> where the three are identified, respectively: 5728, Book 76, Hadith 43; 5734, Book 76, Hadith 49; and 5770, Book 76, Hadith 84. The report of Ibn Kathīr regarding the Prophet's Companion Abū Mūsā al-Ashar'ī is in his *Bidāya*, quoted by Dols in his "Plague in Early Islamic History," p. 378. The quotation from Dols in the same paragraph is also from "Plague in Early Islamic History," p. 378. The words of the caliph 'Umar ibn 'Abd al-'Azīz are from Suyūṭī's *Reports about Plague*, quoted in Dols in "Plague in Early Islamic History," p. 380. The work of Ibn Qutayba has been studies by Jonathan Brown, *Hadith: Muhammad's Legacy in the Medieval and Modern World* (London: Oneworld Publications, 2009). The quotation from Philip Ziegler is from his *The Black Death* (New York: Harper & Row, 1969, p. 92). The words of Hugh Trevor-Roper are lifted from Dols, "Comparative Responses," p. 12. The block quote from Dols is from his "Comparative Responses," p. 6. *The Muslims' Covid-19 Handbook* is to be found at https://jliflc.com/resources/the-muslims-covid-19-handbook-a-guide-on-how-to-deal-with-the-covid-19-pandemic-from-an-islamic-perspective/. Ibn Khaldun has been quoted from his *Muqaddimah*, translated by F. Rosenthal (Princeton NJ: Princeton University Press, 1961, Vol. 1, p. 64. Ibn al-Wardī is quoted in Dols, *Black Death*, p. 114. For Ibn al-Khaṭīb, see Dols, *Black Death*, p. 110.

Viral Corona Capitalism by Vinay Lal

The quotation from William James is from *The Letters of William James, edited by his son Henry James*, 2 vols. (Boston: Atlantic Monthly Press, 1920), Vol 2, p. 259. I have drawn upon the *New York Times* for a number of articles, all from 2020, on the consumer economy during the time of the pandemic, among them Michael Corkery, '"Hero" Raises by Retailers are Fading' (July 15); Peter Eavis, 'Why Not Treat Diversity Like a Profit?' (July 15); Liz Alderman, 'Lockdown Eased, Europe Finds Plenty of Reasons to Shop Again' (July 15); and Sapna Maheshwari, Michael Corkery and Nelson D. Schwartz, 'Consumers Came Back. Is Recovery Sustainable?' (July 17). The conditions at one Amazon Fulfillment Center are described by Emily Guendelsberger in *Time* (18 July 2019). The steps taken by the UK government to provide economic relief are discussed by Richard Partington in *The Guardian* (20 March 2020); for steps taken in India, see *The Wire* (17 May 2020) and *The First Post* (18 May 2020). Work and food insecurity are discussed by Fiona Harvey, 'Coronavirus pandemic will "cause famine of biblical proportions"', *The Guardian* (21 April 2020) and in a report issued by the International Labour Organization, 'Covid-19 and the World of Work', 5th ed. (30 June 2020). Another UN policy brief, 'The Impact of Covid-19 on Women' (9 April 2020) is succinct on the subject indicated by the title, and the quotes are from two articles from *The New Times*: Alisha Haridasani Gupta, 'Why Some Women Call Recession a "Shecession"' (9 May 2020) and Patricia Cohen and Tiffany Hsu, 'Pandemic Could Scar a Generation of Working Mothers' (3 June 2020). On women's participation in the labour force, I have used data from the World Bank: https://data.worldbank.org/indicator/SL.TLF.TOTL.FE.ZS?locations=IN. The implications of the pandemic for the safety and well-being of Indian women are discussed in a *New York Times* article by Kai Schultz and Suhasini Ray (9 June 2020) and the boost to matrimonial online sites in *The New Indian Express* and in *The Hindu*, in articles by Binita Jaiswal and Mini Tejaswi, respectively, both on 25 April 2020. On health spending around the world, see Bradley Sawyer and Cynthia Fox, 'How does health spending in the U.S. compare to other countries?', https://www.healthsystemtracker.org/chart-collection/health-spending-u-s-compare-countries/#item-start (7 December 2018); for Brazil, see Marcia C. Castro et al., 'Brazi's unified health system', *The Lancet* (27 July 2019). Jean Dreze and Amartya Sen, *An Uncertain Glory: India and Its*

Contradictions (London: Allen Lane/Penguin Books, 2013), puts India's shortcomings in the arena of 'development' in perspective with comparisons drawn from Pakistan and Bangladesh, among other countries. On the self-identification with socialism among Americans, see Rana Foroohar, 'American Capitalism's Great Crisis', *Time* (12 May 2016) and Elaine Godfrey, 'Thousands of Americans Have Become Socialists since March', *The Atlantic* (14 May 2020).

Mary Montagu and Ottoman Inoculation by Iftikhar Malik

The extracts from letters are from Mary Wortley Montagu, *Life on the Golden Horn* (Penguin classics, London, 2007). Her other letters appear in *The Turkish Embassy Letters*, edited and annotated by Malcolm Jack & Anita Desai (Virago, London, 2009).

Apart from Richard Knolles, *The General Historie of the Turkes* (Adam Islip, London, 1603), other works on the Turks of this period include: Paul Rycaut, *The History of the Turkish Empire, 1623 to the year 1677* (J. M. for John Starkey, London, 1680); and, Aaron Hill, *A Full and Just Account of the Present State of the Ottoman Empire* (John Mayo, London, 1709).

See also: Isobel Grundy, *Lady Mary Montagu: Comet of the Enlightenment* (OUP, 1999). Her comment about Montagu's fame is from p xvii.

Covid-19, Islam and Pseudoscience by Nidhal Guessoum

Yaqeen Institute's paper can be read at: https://yaqeeninstitute.org/osman-umarji/a-punishment-or-a-mercy-what-we-can-learn-from-the-coronavirus/. Most I`jaz-promoting material, including various statements of the International Commission for Scientific Miracles of the Qur'an and Sunnah, can easily be found on the web, e.g. Abd al-Daim Al-Kaheel's website https://kaheel7.net/. Ahmad Isa Al-Maasarawy's viral tweet is at: https://twitter.com/elmasrw/status/1221177748212854786. Mohamed Elzoghbe's viral video: Corona jundun min junudi-Allah wa indharun khatir ("Corona is a soldier of God and a stern warning") is at: https://www.youtube.com/watch?v=psdTOZzeKL8. Craig Considine's article, from 17 March 2020 issue of *Newsweek*, 'Can the Power of Prayer Alone Stop a Pandemic like the Coronavirus? Even the Prophet Muhammad Thought Otherwise', can be accessed at: https://www.newsweek.com/prophet-prayer-muhammad-covid -19-coronavirus-1492798.

On the criticism of I`jaz, see Ziauddin Sardar, Explorations in Islamic Science (Mansell, London, 1989), Chapter One; Nidhal Guessoum, *Islam's Quantum Question: Reconciling Muslim Tradition and Modern Science*. (I. B. Tauris, London, 2011); "Islam and Science: The next phase of debates", *Zygon*, 50:4, 854-876 2015, and *As'ilatu al-Islam wa al-`Ilm al-Muz`ijah: al-kawn, al-tatawwur, al-i`jaz* (Annoying Questions of Islam and science: the universe, evolution, miraculous content). (Zayed bin Sultan Center, Abu Dhabi, 2017); Stefano Bigliardi, "The "Scientific Miracle of the Qur'an, Pseudoscience, and Conspiracism", *Zygon* 52.1 (2017), 146-171, "The "Scientific Miracle of the Qur'an: Map and Assessment", *Islamic Studies Today: Essays in Honor of Andrew Rippin*. (Brill, Leiden, 2017), , 339-353, and "What We Talk About When We Talk About Iʿjāz", *Social Epistemology Review and Reply Collective* 4.1 (2014), 38-45 2017; Muhammad Atbush, *Naqd al-I`jaz al-`Ilmiy: azmatu al-deen wa al-`ilm* (Critique of Scientific I`jaz: crisis of religion and science) (Masarat Publishers, Kuwait, 2016); .Adnan Zarzour, *al-I`jaz al-`Ilmiy fil Qur'an: dirasatun naqdiyya* (Scientific Miracles in the Qur'an: a critical study) (Dar al-Maqasid, Istanbul, 2018). The quotations from Ibn Khaldun are from *The Muqaddimah: An Introduction to History*, translated by Franz Rosenthal, Princeton and Oxford: Princeton University Press, 1969, 2005), p.387.

Quotes on pseudoscience are from Caleb W. Lack and Jacques Rousseau, *Critical thinking, science, and pseudoscience: why we can't trust our brains*. (New York: Springer, New York, 2016), p. 9 and p35; Scott Lillenfeld 'Foreword: Navigating a Post-Truth World: Ten Enduring Lessons from the Study of Pseudoscience', in *Pseudoscience: The Conspiracy Against Science*, edited by Allison B. Kaufman and James C. Kaufman (MIT Press, Cambridge, Massachusetts , 2018), p. xiv; and David K Hecht, 'Pseudoscience and the Pursuit of Truth', in *Pseudoscience: The Conspiracy Against Science*, edited by Allison B. Kaufman and James C. Kaufman, Cambridge, Massachusetts and London, England: MIT Press, 2018, pp. 3–17.

Swollen Feet by Chandrika Parmar

The SWAN report can be found on their website: http://strandedworkers.in. For Priyanka Shukla stories see: https://www.hindustantimes.com/india-news/in-long-walk-back-home-migrants-battle-hunger-scourge-of-disease/story-TizRfUz69osJQ0Uqmm6jZN.html. The Print story can be found at: https://theprint.in/india/in-covid-19-lockdown-many-of-delhis-poor-and-homeless-are-being-forced-to-starve/389790/?fbclid=IwAR3_HzHSAzoASEwHxvUqfV2ubeeiUrjwnbxhKjhNe5inHrN9NjUCp4_p-zs; Sudarshan Saharkar's article is at: https://ruralindiaonline.org/articles/homeward-bound-through-the-centre-of-india/ and Ipsita Chakravary's piece is at:https://scroll.in/article/963641/a-story-of-swollen-feet-the -physical-toll-of-walking-home-during-lockdown. For Barkha Dutt's columns go to: https://www.hindustantimes.com/columns/barkha-dutt

Most of the other stories mentioned in this article can easily be found online.

Iranian Dilemmas by Lila Randall

Robert Crawford quote appears in Paul Ward and Samantha Meyer, 'Trust, Social Quality and Wellbeing: A Sociological Exegesis', Development and Society 38 (2) 339-363 2009; https://www.jstor.org/stable/deveandsoci.38.2.339. On the lack of trust on the government, see:
https://www.dw.com/en/coronavirus-iranians-lose-trust-in-government-as-virus-spreads/a-52651804. On censorship in Iran, see: https://www.indexoncensorship.org/2009/01/iran-thirty-years-on/

Viral Dreams by Leyla Jagiella

The poem appears in *Diwan of Ali ibn Abi Talib* translated by Abdullah Ayaz Mullanee, which can be viewed at https://www.mnblind.org/pdf/18-arabic-grammar/8537-15-diwan-ali-ml-ayaz-mullaanee/file?fbclid=IwAR1iye7EbvoJAeIpfN2NG8KhWlIP9pEWYiMvSTNINq3XwWNhT1L_3Z-51UU

The *Scientific American* article on pandemic dreams can be read at: https://www.scientificamerican.com/article/the-covid-19-pandemic-is-changing-our-dreams/

Existential Terror by James Brooks

An excellent BBC film about the BSE scandal, *Mad Cow Disease: The Great British Beef Scandal*, directed by Will Lorimer, is available at https://www.bitchute.com/video/FTmBU5VykG8a/

The *Independent* article, 'Victims face insanity and certain death' by Jojo *Moyes* of 21 March 1996 can be found at: https://bit.ly/3mNPRpB. The full transcript of *12 Monkeys* can be found on a fansite: https://bit.ly/3053Iyd. Philip Larkin's poem, *Aubade* is on the Poetry Foundation website: https://bit.ly/3j0y4tk; *Flight from Death: The Quest for Immortality* is a 2003 documentary film by Patrick Shen about

Ernest Becker's ideas and the related experimental work of Jeff Greenberg, Sheldon Solomon and Tom Pyszczynski. It is available on YouTube: https://bit.ly/33S0Hm6; and the BMJ paper, 'Spiritual dimensions of dying in pluralist societies' by Liz Grant, Scott A Murray, Aziz Sheikh, 16 September 2010, can be found at: https://doi.org/10.1136/bmj.c4859

Elements of Conviviality by Peter Coates

The quote from Rom Harré is from his article, 'Ontology and Science', *Beshara Magazine*, issue 3 8-15, 1987; and the Junayd quote is taken from Ibn Arabi's *The Wisdom of the Prophets*, translated by Titus Burckardt and Angela Culme-Seymour (Beshara Publications, Cheltenham, 1975) p131. See also: Seyyed Hossein Nasr, *The Encounter of Man and Nature* (Allen and Unwin, London, 1968); Ali Hassan Abdel-Kader, *Life, Personality and Writings of al-Junayd* (Islamic Book Trust, Oxford, 2013); and Peter Coates, *Ibn Arabi and Modern Thought* (Anqa Publications, Oxford, 2002).

White Muslims by Josef Linnhoff

For Leon Moosavi's account of the 're-racialisation' of white Muslims, see 'White Privilege in the Lives of Muslim Converts in Britain', *Ethnic and Racial Studies* 38 (11); 1918 – 1933, and 'The Racialisation of Muslim Converts in Britain and their experiences of Islamophobia', *Critical Sociology* 41 (1); 41-56. For Esra Ozyurek's study on ethnic German Muslims, see *Being German, Becoming Muslim: Race, Religion and Conversion in New Europe* (Princeton, New Jersey: Princeton University Press, 2015).

On Cognitive Immunity by Ebrahim Moosa

Works referred to in this essay include: Ibn Sina, *Al-Qānūn Fī 'l-Ṭibb. 2 ed. 3 vols (Dār al-Kutub al-'Ilmīya*, Beirut, 2009); William H Calvin, *A Brief History of the Mind: From Apes to Intellect and Beyond* (OUP, 2004); Priscilla Wald, *Contagious: Cultures, Carriers, and the Outbreak Narrative* (Duke University Press, Durham NC, 2008) and Marina Gorbis, 'To Protect Democracy We Need to IUpgrade Our Cognitive Immunity' in *Medium* 2020.

The quotes form Carl Sagan are from his *The Demon-Haunted World* (Random House, New York, 1996), p94.

CONTRIBUTORS

Uzmah Ali is working on her first novel, her debut poetry collection is published by Waterloo Press ● **James Brooks** is a science journalist and writer ● **Peter Coates**, former Senior Lecturer in Philosophy, Department of Psychology, University of Lincoln, is the author of *Ibn Arabi and Modern Thought* ● **Nidhal Guessoum** is Professor of Astrophysics at American University of Sharjah, UAE ● **Syed Nomanul Haq** is Dean, Institute of Liberal Arts, University of Management and Technology, Lahore ● **Usama Hasan** is senior researcher in Islamic Studies at the Quilliam Foundation, London ● **Anwar Ibrahim**, Malaysian politician, is President of People's Justice Party and Leader of Opposition ● **Leyla Jagiella** is a cultural anthropologist exploring orthodoxy and heterodoxy in South Asian Islam ● **Vinay Lal**, Professor of History at UCLA, is the author of *The Fury of Covid-19* ● **Josef Linnhoff** is Director of Editorial at the Usuli Institute, Los Angeles ● **Nazik al-Malaika** is a well-known Iraqi poet ● **Iftikhar Malik** is Professor of History at Bath Spa University ● **Ehsan Masood**, a science journalist, is a leader writer for *Nature* ● **Sara Mohr** is a PhD candidate in Assyriology at Brown University's Department of Egyptology and Assyriology ● **Ebrahim Moosa** is Mirza Family Professor of Islamic Thought and Muslim Societies, University of Notre Dame ● **Chandrika Parmar** is faculty member at S P Jain Institute of Management and Research, Mumbai ● **Samia Rahman** is Director of the Muslim Institute ● **Lila Randall** is a science journalist ● **Carol Rumens** is an award-winning British poet ● **Osama Siddique** is the author of *Pakistan's Experience with Formal Law: An Alien Justice* and the historical novel, *Snuffing Out the Moon* ● **Colin Tudge**, biologist and writer, is co-founder of the College for Rural Farming and Food Culture, and author of *The Great Rethink*.